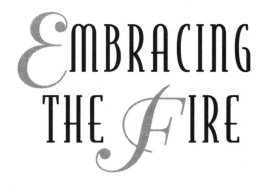

EMBRACING THE FIRE

ALSO BY JULIA A. BOYD

In the Company of My Sisters

Girlfriend to Girlfriend

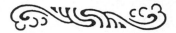

EMBRACING THE FIRE

SISTERS TALK ABOUT SEX AND RELATIONSHIPS

JULIA A. BOYD

A DUTTON BOOK

DUTTON
Published by the Penguin Group
Penguin Books USA Inc., 375 Hudson Street,
New York, New York 10014, U.S.A.
Penguin Books Ltd, 27 Wrights Lane,
London W8 5TZ, England
Penguin Books Australia Ltd, Ringwood,
Victoria, Australia
Penguin Books Canada Ltd, 10 Alcorn Avenue,
Toronto, Ontario, Canada M4V 3B2
Penguin Books (N.Z.) Ltd, 182–190 Wairau Road,
Auckland 10, New Zealand

Penguin Books Ltd, Registered Offices:
Harmondsworth, Middlesex, England

First published by Dutton, an imprint of Dutton Signet, a division of
Penguin Books USA Inc.
Distributed in Canada by McClelland & Stewart Inc.

First Printing, February, 1997
10 9 8 7 6 5 4 3 2 1

REGISTERED TRADEMARK—MARCA REGISTRADA

ISBN 0-525-93959-8
CIP data is available.

Printed in the United States of America
Set in Stone Informal
Designed by Stanley S. Drate/Folio Graphics Co. Inc.

This book is printed on acid-free paper. ⊗

To Momi
Lavada Conyers (1924–1994)
and
To Mama
Annie Dunn (1908–1995)

There aren't words enough to express my love.
Your lessons will always remain in my heart.

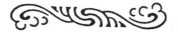

ACKNOWLEDGMENTS

This book was truly a labor of love: I labored over every word of it and love all of you who stood by me in the creative process. I would like to thank my family—the Conyers, Dunns, and Boyds—for your love, support and encouragement; I'm truly blessed to have you all in my life. To my son, Michael, my greatest love, I'm so proud of you and all that you've accomplished. Jung Hur, I love you, li'l girl; thanks for being my workout and shopping buddy. My agent, Elizabeth Wales, I'm proud to have you as my agent and girlfriend—we'll go on that nature walk real soon, as long as it's on a sunny beach somewhere in the South Pacific. To my editor, Carole DeSanti, thank you doesn't begin to say it all, but that's where I'll start; I'm so fortunate to have you as my editor and friend; your ability and talent to help authors such as myself to shape dreams into words is truly a gift, and you do it well; thank you from the bottom of my heart. To Alex Swenson, Carole's assistant, thanks for your steady support and encouragement. To Marsha Leslie, girlfriend, I really appreciate all the time and energy you put into editing the first draft of this manuscript. Zola Mumford, my assistant, you've been a lifesaver in the past year; thanks for being my second pair of eyes and ears and keeping me on track. To that bodacious crew of sexy divas I call girlfriends—Charlotte "I can't believe you said that" Watson Sherman, Carletta Wilson, Colleen "Too Sexy for Words" McElroy, Amy Laly, Perviz, Faith Davis, Alma Arnold, Gail "Where Are My Car Keys?" Myers, Marilyn Fullen-Collins, Dr. Marion "Go 'Head, Girlfriend" Rock, Barbara Thomas, Jody Kim, Fran Frazier, Libby Rand, Cheyla Axtell, Donna Manier, Alma Adams, Bev "Hey Girl" Williaby, and Alice Snyder—I couldn't have done this book without your continued love, support, and incredible patience; I love you all. To Karen Horn, Lisha, Karen Black, Alpha, and Charles, thank you all for feeding me, making me laugh, and lifting my spirits on my weekly visits to the shop. To Nori "Li'l Bit" Balderas, Michelle "Miss Attitude" Brake, Irene "Sassy" Bertucci, Brenda "Don't You See Grown Folks Talk'n" Freeman, Rachel "Smily" Warrick, Lisa "How May I Assist You?" Goings, Kathrina "Clean Desk" Sharman, Stephanie Jordan, and Gary Weiss—thanks for helping me keep my head above water and helping me to laugh. And to the rest of my Group Health Cooperative family, thanks for your continued support. To John "J.B." Krause, thank you for your kindness and support. I would also like to send out a very special thanks to all of the sisters who contributed to this project.

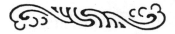

CONTENTS

Contents

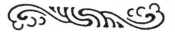

INTRODUCTION

The idea for this book evolved from a two-hour telephone conversation with one of my close sister friends. She had just broken up with her partner of two years and needed a sympathetic ear. "I wish I knew what a normal, healthy relationship looked like," she stated soberly.

"Why can't I have a decent relationship? I don't think it's asking too much to want satisfying sex and a loving relationship in the same package. I know that life doesn't come with a book of instructions, but I would like to have just one relationship work out right." She went on to catalog a host of conflicting fears, desires, and expectations. "Every time I think I've got it right something goes wrong. Maybe if I wasn't my mother's daughter, I wouldn't believe that I had to settle for one and wish for the other. But I guess I'm too much like Mama to expect that things can be different for me. I don't know, sis, maybe it's just me; do you think I expect too much?"

As I listened I found myself slowly reviewing all the messages that I had received over the years concerning sex and relationships. Forty-plus years, one divorce, and one grown child later I, along with my sister friend, shared the dilemma of continually grappling with the emotional baggage we were carrying about being sexual adults.

Hearing my sister friend's hurt and confusion reminded me of the messages many of us carried from childhood to adulthood. Parents and other well-meaning adults emotionally bound us to beliefs and expectations that rarely fit the journeys we often found ourselves taking. As adolescents we listened dutifully to messages about sex that were more often than not coded and indirect, pointed pieces of communication intended to steer our future behavior. These messages often took the form of stern warnings:

"If you get pregnant I'll . . ."

"Don't be thinkin' you're gonna be droppin' your problems on this here doorstep. . . ."

"If you don't watch yourself, you're gonna end up like . . ."

"Hazel had to send that girl away, 'cause she got herself in trouble."

And pronouncements from the pulpit:

"And the Holy Book says fornication and all acts of uncleanness outside of marriage are a sin against God."

"Wives, submit yourselves only unto your husbands."

"Just remember, ain't no man gonna buy a cow when he can get the milk for free."

"Don't be so fast. Leave those li'l boys alone. There'll

2

be plenty enough time for that sort of stuff when you're grown."

These last two were the coded messages I received from my mother, who believed that as I became older, I also would become wiser and reach a magic place of discovery in the sex-and-relationship department. Well, I became older but the magic didn't happen—not in the way that my mother believed or hoped that it would happen.

I grew up believing that my life would look something like my mother's. After all, I reasoned to myself, Momi wouldn't lie to me; she knew the ropes. I had only to look at her life as proof positive of that fact. Her loving long-term marriage, well-cared-for children, warm, loving home—all the ingredients of stable domesticity were part of my expectations. What I didn't learn until much later is that Momi's map didn't fit my own life journey. Our parents and the other adults in our lives meant well in their teachings, but the indirect messages we received were confusing because they were wrapped in parental fear and distrust.

The turning point in my personal journey came after my divorce—however, in listening to many of my sister friends' experiences, I recognize that their personal catalysts for life changes have happened through a variety of circumstances: the birth of a child, the decision not to have children, building a new career, returning to school, starting a new relationship, leaving an old relationship, children leaving home, the death of a parent, onset of menopause, etc. The stories of why and how we change at different points in our lives are as individual and diverse as our voices. In sharing our stories we have discovered that we are women who enjoy being sexual. We have taken comfort in discovering that we aren't alone in wanting to have long-term and short-term relationships and one-night stands. We have encouraged one another to have fun with sex by talking openly about our wants, needs, and desires sexually and in relationships. We have supported one another in talking to our children about the realities of sex and relationships. As sister friends we have found strength in ourselves and each other by sharing our stories. We have found that there isn't a right or wrong way to sexual or relationship fulfillment; there are just life experiences that give us all a backdrop for learning how to define our individual preferences.

I never heard my mother say the word *sex*. She, like the majority of women of her era, viewed s-e-x (Momi would sometimes spell words she couldn't bring herself to say) as being directly linked to "marital relations," and in her mind there were only two types of women who engaged in sex: "married women" and "bad women." Married women had husbands, raised children, and settled down; bad women were often referred to as "shameless hussies" (harsher terms were used out of our earshot); they chased men, did nasty things, and often had children by different men.

I still remember being in the sixth grade and running home from school at breakneck speed, slamming the door behind me, and yelling for a dictionary.

"Girl, what in the world is wrong with you running

in the house like that, making all that noise?" my mother asked in an irritated voice.

"Momi, quick, I need a dictionary. Where is it?" I asked breathlessly.

"It's in the bookcase, where it always is," Momi quietly responded as she laid my baby brother down in the bassinet for his nap. "What in the world are you looking up now?" she asked as she watched me hurriedly scan the shelves, looking for the huge black Webster's dictionary.

"Eric Newton called Shirley Jenkins a 'ho' today at recess. And when Shirley told Miss Brown, Miss Brown made Eric stand against the wall. And then Miss Brown said we shouldn't use words when we didn't know what they mean. When Shirley asked her what *ho* meant, Miss Brown said we should go home and look it up in the dictionary. So I'm looking it up." I explained this in a rambling tone as I flipped through page after page of the dictionary. "Momi, how do you spell *ho*?"

"Girl, close that book and carry yourself on outside and play." But being determined not to be put off, I persisted. "Momi, what is a ho? I can't find it!"

"It's a woman that does nasty things with her body. Now get on outside and play before I find some work round here for you to do." My mother's tone of voice told me that she was clearly uncomfortable with the topic. We didn't talk about such things as "bad women" in our house. It was believed that talking about "those types of things" might put ideas in our heads. And my mother was very invested in her role as a good mother who believed it was her duty to raise "good girls": girls who would grow up, become "good" women, marry, and settle down. I can still hear her question of "Girl, when are you going to settle down?" a year after my divorce, when I told her I had met someone I liked.

"Settle down and do what, Momi?" I teased.

"You know good and well what I'm talking about," she replied, sounding just a tad miffed. She was right. I did know what she was talking about, but I also knew she wouldn't say it. My mother was afraid that I would become a "bad woman." After all, the signs were there—I was divorced, had a child, and was going out with men. What I wanted to tell my mother but didn't was that her life experiences (marriage and family were my mother's life) didn't fit my needs in the area of sex and relationships. I also recognized that my mother, like her mother before her, didn't have the language or knowledge that I had acquired as an adult. My mother was giving me what information she had, and again like many of the women of her era, what she had was based on experiences either she or someone she knew had undergone.

"Relationships can be tricky and I don't want you to be hurt, so just watch yourself."

"You're going to experience emotional feelings and attractions that may seem overwhelming at times—be careful."

These are the messages I believe our parents wanted to give us, but timing, language, fears, and often their own experiences got in the way. Like my sister friend, I had tried to follow my mother's messages for having a relationship and they didn't fit, so I had to travel a different path.

Embracing the Fire is based on my struggle to discover and accept the fact that the messages about sex and relationships I'd received as a young woman didn't necessarily fit my—nor many of my sisters'—life experiences. First, finding my voice as a woman led me to a place of personal pain (divorce) and confusing freedom as I tried to navigate the world of relationships based on an outdated emotional road map. Then, as I listened to my sister friend express her own confusion, I realized that as Black women we all shared generational baggage that often caused us to stumble when we tried to take a new path. *"What I want is a normal healthy relationship"* or *"I'm not ready for a relationship right now, but I don't want to give up sex"* is what I have often heard from sisters who find themselves navigating the stormy waters of intimate relationships.

With *Embracing the Fire*, it is my hope to encourage us to talk more openly and honestly sister to sister, mother to daughter and son, and lover to lover about the realities of our lives. *Embracing the Fire* grew out of my concern that we were only seeing, hearing, and reading about the war stories, tragedies, and misinformation often associated with our intimate lives. I also want to help sisters decode some of the messages that we've been given from our mothers and other well-meaning adults. My fear is that we might forget why we choose to be continually sexually active despite the war stories—because we enjoy the pleasure and mystery of it all. I want *Embracing the Fire* to fling open the doors of communication as we share our sexual dreams, fantasies, experiences, fears, hopes, and desires in an area that needs the presence of our voices as Black women. We are, in many cases, choosing to travel paths that look decidedly different from the paths our mothers took in life. It's my hope that this book will help us to struggle less and share more meaningful communication with our younger sisters and brothers about sexual experiences. I believe it's important that our younger sisters and brothers learn from us as adults that being sexual is more than just a physical matter. It is, in essence, our ability to communicate how much we love and embrace our sense of self and our differences emotionally, physically, and spiritually. Most of all I want *Embracing the Fire* to be a celebration of who we are as sensuous Black women.

So throw your baggage in the trunk and slide into the front seat—we've got some items to pick up on our journey.

Because of privacy and out of respect for those sisters who were gracious enough to share their stories with me, names and identities of individuals have been changed.

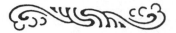

THE BAGGAGE
WE CARRY

I've been dreaming about sex again. My long, sensuous legs are wrapped around the hard waist of some gorgeous bronze hunk; our arms intertwine as sweat-slicked bodies melt together and move to the rhythm of our swelling passion. . . . And then my alarm goes off, fading my dream lover into the sounds of the early-morning traffic report.

I've been dreaming about sex a lot lately. I'm really not surprised—it's been six months since my relationship ended, and with these dreams my sensual senses are starting to reawaken. As much as I hate breakups, I've become familiar with my style of coping: one month of pitiful helplessness, crying and feeling totally lost; one month of rehashing every word ever spoken between us and endlessly analyzing everything I thought went wrong; one month of anger bordering on rage (at the injustice of his leaving); one month of congratulating myself for making it through the first three without having a nervous breakdown;

and two more of throwing myself deeply into my work and thoroughly convincing myself that any relationship of mine was bound to fail. I know myself well enough to recognize that in the first three months this process starts out an emotional explosion spilling over onto any and all parts of my everyday life, and it ends with a cooling down in the last three to form a cold steel blanket of emotional numbness. Feelings of a sexual nature are the first to go and the last to return, with other emotional feelings sandwiched in between. My dreams of sex told me I was right on schedule emotionally, and as much as I dreaded the memories of what I had lost—the passionate embraces, the deep, sensuous kisses, and the teasing touch—I welcomed the emotional sexual release. My sexual dreams allowed my body to remember what my waking mind wanted to forget . . . I am a sensual woman who enjoys the pleasures of having a healthy sexual appetite.

I've noticed that my dreams about sex flow much smoother after a period of emotional hibernation, and I've noticed that it feels safer to dream about sex than to have it in real life because I don't have to handle the waking realities of managing a relationship and the baggage that entails. I also don't have to consciously struggle with the myths ("Black women are uptight and prudish about sexual matters") and taboos ("Nice girls don't talk about such things") that demonized my early years. While as an adult I've long felt that I've outgrown the stereotypical typecasting of who and what a sexual Black woman is or should be—cold, aloof, hot to trot, animal in bed, prudish, or unimaginative—I occasionally hear my mother's constant warnings "not to be fast, or act too womanish" whenever I seek to feed my sexual hunger with some- one new. In my dreams I flirt, tease, and aim to get sexually pleased and no one cares one way or another how womanish or fast I behave. Dreams allow me to cut loose and become the wild sexual Black woman who defies all the myths and stereotypical images, and Momi's warnings are forgotten, replaced with my wanton pleasure. The problem I encounter is that my dream images rarely if ever spill over into my waking sexual reality without the residue of guilt attached. Without my really recognizing it, my mother's teach- ings about proper ladylike etiquette packed my emo- tional suitcases to the top, and the relaxed freedom of sexual pleasure is securely folded, tucked and hidden on the bottom of the pile.

At age sixteen I had a huge crush on my best friend's older brother. Jason was six-one, slender with the well- defined muscled body that led our high school basket- ball team to the state finals. His deep olive complex- ion, coal black eyes, and sexy handsome smile had every girl in school drooling, and I was at the head of the pack. There was only one problem: Jason had a girlfriend, Rita, also a good friend of mine, and they were crazy about each other. As far as I was concerned Jason was Adonis and in my diary I was his Aphrodite, but in the real world he considered me no more than a kid sister. Every night I dreamed about Jason, how we would run away together, get married, and live happily ever after in a place of endless love. I faith- fully recorded my dreams in my diary, painstakingly recording every detail of our future lives together, how he would call me sweetheart, and the warm moistness of his kisses, how I would fix his favorite meals (this was a fantasy, remember), and we would feed each other from our plates as we lay in bed and would then make passionate love. Momi discovered my diary, as mothers who are major housecleaners tend to do, and in what I'm sure she felt was a casual conversation reminded me that Jason had a girlfriend.

"You're much too young to be thinking 'bout boys. Keep your head in your books and make something of yourself. I've told you before, being fast will only lead you into trouble. Besides, that boy's got a girlfriend—I thought I taught you better than that." I was crushed, hurt, angry, and ashamed and responded in my best sixteen-year-old indignant voice.

"How could you read my diary? And besides, it's no big deal. They're only dreams anyway."

"When you get your own house, you can write and do whatever you please, but in this house everything is open to inspection and don't you forget it. What do you know 'bout makin' love anyway? I've told you a million times 'bout being fast. You'll be grown soon enough, and till that time comes you keep your head in your books and leave dreamin' 'bout these little boys alone. Mark my words, those kind of dreams only lead to trouble, and I don't intend to have you bringin' that kind of trouble in here, you understand?"

I understood perfectly. I understood that feelings of a sexual nature were to be ignored, erased without a trace of expression. But what Momi didn't understand was that my dreams belonged to me, and while I could successfully hide my feelings during my waking moments, my unconscious dream state was an unruly child that refused to cooperate. I didn't give up dreaming about Jason; I just stopped writing down my fantasies. And just as Momi had ignored my question about reading my diary, I chose to ignore her question about my knowledge of making love. Of course I didn't have any real knowledge on the subject—we didn't discuss such things at our house, outside of the cursory "You'll know when it happens," or "you'll be grown soon enough and you'll find out then" responses that met my inquiries on the subject. Of course, I thought I knew everything about everything. At sixteen, growing up in the wholesome, clean suburb of Fair Oaks, California, in 1967, I knew pretty much what every other teenager in my community knew about sex . . . nothing. We double- and triple-dated, if they could actually be called dates, thereby severely limiting our chances of doing any more than kissing, and even that happened with our lips securely closed for fear of breaching some unspoken moral code. Our parents knew one another and frequently socialized together at church, school, and community functions, so chances of any of us kids getting out of line were pretty remote. What I knew of sex I learned from reading trashy novels that my girlfriends passed around in the locker room at school. The good stuff was double underlined and the best pages were raggedy from dog-eared marking, and even then most of the so-called hot scenes only talked about heaving bosoms and long fiery passionate kisses. Since I didn't have enough bosom to heave, and it was hard to get fired

up or passionate with closed lips, my mother needn't
have worried about me getting into any kind of sexual
trouble.

As an adult I have a much clearer understanding of
my mother's worry and concerns. After all, at sixteen
my mother was married and had my oldest brother. I
heard the stories about her early years with my father
and how hard it was for them to scratch out a living
while raising a family and still being so young themselves. I also got the lectures that always began with
the warning about "being fast" whenever I begged to
stay out later, or attend unchaperoned events. "Stop
tryin' to be so fast, you'll have plenty of time for those
things when you're older" was what I heard whenever
I complained. My mother didn't tell me about sex or
making love, as much as she warned, and tried to protect me from it. She believed her messages of "not
being fast or womanish" would keep me from repeat-
ing any mistakes she might have made growing up.

"I was lucky," she would emphasize. "I got a good
man who wanted to be with me. We loved each other
enough to struggle and make it through the hard
times." To me her messages sounded old-fashioned
and intrusive. After all, what could she possibly know
about being sixteen, having crushes, being in love,
and—for that matter—sex. She and Daddy had been
married forever, and surely, I reasoned in my sixteen-
year-old mind, as a grown-up my mother couldn't re-
late to my world. I didn't want to believe that my
mother understood my dreams of romantic desire because it would have meant that I was more like her
than I could comfortably tolerate. Somewhere in the

recesses of my mind I knew that she and Daddy loved each other, but it was different, it had to be. I wanted to believe their love for each other was born of duty, not passion. At sixteen I wanted to ignore my mother's flirtatious manner with my father, and his affection-ate endearments to her. I wanted to deny their warmth toward each other, because I was sixteen and sorely needed to have these feelings of emotional attraction that I felt to be my own. What I forgot to factor into my teenage logic was that my mother as a woman had been there (sixteen) and done that (shared similar dreams), and she did have wisdom that I needed, even though her wisdom was enclosed in her fears for me. I didn't hear her dreams when she told me stories about her and Daddy, I only heard her fears of what my life could end up being if I followed in her footsteps.

I heard the stories, especially after the discovery of my diary, but what I saw in their relationship was somewhat different. My parents had a loving mar-riage and I witnessed their love daily, providing me with tangible evidence that my mother's warning of "being fast" wouldn't necessarily lead me in the wrong direction. Seeing my mother embrace the fire in her life, the one she continually warned me about as being much too hot, and living out her dream, ac-tively encouraged me to do the same with my dreams. On some level I knew that I had to take Momi's warn-ing to heart, and outwardly, at least for a time, I smothered my passions, waiting for that magical time of being old enough. But there was a part of me, my dreams that weren't touched as deeply by my mother's fears, and in the privacy of my own thoughts I got to unpack the sexual fears and play with the feelings that she had so carefully and in her own loving way packed for me. I'm not always sure how I did it or really when I chose to start pushing past my mother's unspoken boundaries regarding making love or being a sexual Black woman in my own right, but the magic time of being grown and taking emotional risks did occur, and I started digging around in my bags and trying on certain emotional behaviors of a sexual nature during the light of day.

In my eighth year of marriage, at the ripe age of twenty-eight, after the majority of excitement and bliss of being a newlywed had long since worn off, my then-husband and I were making long-term career choices. He had been working at a Fortune 500 company for about a year when he received a promotion that meant moving to Washington State. The decision to move was an emotional one for me. It meant leaving my family, to whom I was extremely close, and some of my oldest and dearest friends. As always, my first line of comfort was Momi.

"How did you do it, Momi? How did you have the courage to leave your family and friends when Daddy had to make moves for business?"

"Baby, you just do what you have to do. Your father had to work, and as far as I was concerned him and you kids were the only family I needed to be worried about. It ain't like you're moving to the other side of the world; Daddy said that Seattle is only a day-and-a-half drive from Stockton, so you know we'll be up to visit and you all can come down here for vacations."

"It's just going to be so different—who will I talk to?" I moaned.

"You just remember that your husband and baby are your first priority now. That boy's got a good job, and a chance to make it. Moving is a small price to pay," Momi stated in a firm stern voice. "And besides," she added in a softer tone, "you know we'll always be here for you."

So after a host of congratulatory bon voyage parties, we made our move to Seattle, Washington. The first six months were wonderful. Moving into our house and getting to know our community provided us with time together that we both enjoyed. The newness of everything also seemed to rejuvenate our sexual feelings for each other. But I noticed that after that period of adjustment, we again fell into a routine that looked and felt all too familiar. He was working all the time and I was still looking to him to supply all of my needs: husband, lover, and friend.

In the beginning I chalked it up to the pressures of the move, but as the weeks turned into months I noticed that not only were we hardly speaking to each other; our enjoyment of sexual intimacy had all but disappeared too. A year after our move Momi and Daddy came to visit us in Seattle for the first time. I had hoped that their visit would lessen some of the tension between us but it seemed to strain our relationship even further. One night Momi and I were in the kitchen making dinner and I mentioned that I was feeling sexually numb. "I don't know, Momi, sex just doesn't feel or seem as exciting as it used to be," I said, and then with just a twinge of hesitation I asked, "Am

I normal? Is it normal to want sex to be more exciting?"

My mother's eyes met mine as she momentarily stopped stirring the corn-bread batter. It was a fleeting but telling glance, one that I remembered from childhood that silently told me she would listen and then give me her pat answer.

"Ain't nothing wrong with you, baby. That's just part of life. Now turn the oven on so it can start heatin' up." This was her polite way of ending any further conversation on the subject. She didn't tell me, but somehow I read it in her response that she felt that I was somehow wanting to "be fast" sexually, and she was right. Without really answering directly, my mother had given me unspoken permission to allow my sexual numbness to remain in place. Still, I wanted what I had in the beginning of my marriage, the freshness and passion of sexual discovery. I wanted the feisty enjoyment of hearing my husband moan with pleasure, and laughing complaints that I was wearing him out in bed. I wanted to be excited again at watching him come out of a hot steamy shower with a towel wrapped around his waist. I wanted and needed him to show me that he noticed and missed my sense of sexual excitement, but he seemed in a sexual rut too. I wondered if he shared my feelings of being sexually lost, and grew tired of replacing passion with routine movements that looked sexual but felt totally empty. I wondered but I never asked him, because it felt too much like one more wedge that would come between us. I didn't like feeling sexually numb, empty, and withdrawn; I wanted to feel what I believed was sexually normal, but things between us never reached a stage of recovery.

A couple of years later when I called to tell Momi that my husband and I were getting a divorce, she asked anxiously if there was another woman in his life. I knew she was thinking about our previous conversation when I told her about feeling sexually numb. I did what I felt I needed to do to protect her—I lied and said no. I knew my mother wondered, and being a lot like her in genetic makeup, I wondered and worried too. Were my ex-husband's reasons for choosing someone else somehow linked to sexual inadequacy on my part? At one point in our separation I actually asked him and he said no, but during that time in our lives I wasn't real willing to believe or trust anything he told me. Was it normal for me to feel sexually numb or bored at times? Did Momi experience this numbness in her relationship with Daddy? Was dreaming and fantasizing about "being (sexually) fast" normal? Maybe I wasn't fast or womanish enough to hold on to a man, any man, even my husband; what had I done wrong? Was Momi keeping sexual secrets from me? I had lots of questions without answers and I wasn't ready to believe that what I wanted to know about myself sexually was "just a part of life." My divorce forced me to ask myself these questions and at the same time I recognized that I had to examine some of the larger, more complex issues surrounding my beliefs, practices, needs, and wants about being a sexual Black woman in today's world.

Before I fully understood my six-month period of relationship breakup recovery, I found myself becoming obsessed with the phrase "sexually normal." Was I normal in the sex department? What the hell was normal anyway? Clearly Momi's answer that my feeling shutdown was "just a part of life" only served to fuel my anxiety instead of bringing me to a state of comfortable reassurance, as she had hoped. I found myself doing odd little things like studying the observable postures of other women I encountered on a day-to-day basis, wondering and trying to magically detect if they also struggled with the whole concept of being sexually normal. I cringed inwardly and changed hairdressers after hearing one of the stylists comment, after a particularly difficult customer had left the salon, that she hoped that woman would hurry up and find a man and "get her a li'l piece" 'cause she was driving her crazy with all of her foolishness. I watched couples shopping together in the supermarket, silently speculating to myself about whether or not they had normal sex lives. It seemed the more I searched for an example of "sexually normal," the less I found to conquer my own fears.

Sis, did you ever stop to think that what you were going through was normal? I went through all that same stuff when I broke up with my first husband, and when I divorced my second husband I went through it again; that's when I really knew it was normal.

Gracie

Well, it might be normal for you two, but the only thing I went through when I left that fool I was with some years back was my checkbook. And, honey, I went through that much too quickly.

Queenie

I understand now that what I was experiencing was sexually normal, but at that time the lack of sexual feelings really scared me. My ex-husband was my first sexual partner, so I didn't have anything to compare my feelings with or against. I was very Catholic in those days and like my parents, who were my only role models, I took my marriage vows very seriously.

Well, I've never been married, but I experience those feelings too. It's like you said, sometimes I get so wrapped up in my work until I forget all about sex. And then there are times when I get so horny till everything I see resembles a penis, but I just wait it out, 'cause I know those feelings are gonna pass; they always do.

Ella

I don't think about sex or not think about sex, so I can't speak to feeling sexually numb. I do know that when the urge strikes me and I don't have a special somebody at the moment, I just take matters into my own hands so to speak. I wasn't really raised to believe that you had to be married in order to have sex, so it's never really bothered me one way or the other.

Zoey

My mother is still buggin' me about marrying De-Wayne. I'm so tired of hearing "That's a good man you got there. I don't see why you don't go on ahead and marry him and settle down. Arletta needs a daddy, and he's good to her too. You gonna keep on and some woman's gonna come along and snatch him right out from under you." I keep telling her that we're not ready to take that step just yet. Arletta has a daddy, and, yes, DeWayne is good to both of us, but I'm good to him too. Mama's so busy wondering what everyone is sayin' about us, especially her church sisters, till she just can't hear what I'm saying. So I've just given up sayin' anything. I ain't in no hurry and neither is DeWayne. I know that road you're talkin' about sis, I've been down it once myself, and as far as I'm concerned once is one time too many. I'd rather have one good man than dream about what kind of man I could have.

Jonie

This may sound silly but even though Leon and I have been married twenty years this spring, and I confess I love him dearly, there are times when I can't stand the sight, smell, or touch of him. And I'll admit I do fantasize about what it would be like to be with someone else. Deep down inside I know I'd never do it, but it's fun sometimes to just think about it. I'm like Zoey, I don't know if it's normal or not, and I can't really say that I feel sexually numb, but it happens sometimes. Like I said, I love Leon and I'm committed to our relationship, so I know I wouldn't act on my fantasies, but it's fun to have them sometimes.

Cyree

The Baggage We Carry

Do you ever tell Leon about your fantasy, Cyree?

Nonie

No child! I said I fantasize. I didn't say I went crazy.

Cyree

Well before Winyah came along, I thought I was totally burned out and fed up with men period. I wasn't numb. I was just mad as hell and determined not to take any more stuff off of anybody. I wasn't like you, sis, in that when I looked at a couple all I could think about was how much stuff the woman had to be puttin' up with in order to have a man in her life. The only thing my mama packed in my emotional suitcase, as you say, is good sense, and I was gonna use it all. Winyah will be the first to tell you that it really took a while for me to let him in the door, and even now we go toe to toe and head to head on some things, but I've let my guard down enough to trust him and so far we've been married fifteen years.

Roxy

How did you come to grips with your issues, sis? When did you figure out that all those things you went through were sexually normal?

Ella

To be real honest, Ella, I'm still struggling with some of my sexual demons. The only real solid thing that I've learned about sex is that there is no such thing as normal; everybody has her own process for dealing with being sexual or not being sexual, as the case may be. It's taken me years to figure out just one small part of my process for dealing with sexual issues. Every time I get into a relationship and it doesn't work out, I'm tempted to just throw in the towel. I slide into my old feeling of sexual numbness like a pair of worn-out house shoes. I know I could stay in those house shoes forever, but at some point those house shoes are going to become uncomfortable too. Like Roxy I'm going to have to be willing to take a risk and be willing to confront my feelings. I'm learning that it's okay to have and not run away from scary feelings like sexual numbness, because feelings don't last forever, and being sexually numb is no exception to the rule. The thing that's helped me the most has been talking to people I trust and who care about me. Talking to all of you has helped me feel less alone. I've found that I'm not the only one to dream or fantasize about sex, feel numb, get angry, or have emotional baggage from my mother. Recently I discovered that I can feel just as sexually vulnerable in a relationship as I do when I'm not in a relationship. The reason I may feel sexually vulnerable in a relationship may be different, but the feeling is the same.

I'm finding that as I go through different phases of my womanhood, I learn new and different things about myself emotionally, physically, and sexually. For example, when I was younger I wanted to be chosen; it was important for guys to see me as sexually attractive. As an adult I'm discovering that it's more important for me to define my own sense of sexual attractiveness. However, there are still times when I continue to struggle with this issue. I think the most important lesson I've learned regarding my sexual nature is that I don't have to be afraid, because I'm not alone in my learning process: we're all learning together.

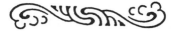

IN THE MIRROR

"Do you think I'm fat?" The words were out before I could stop them. The question I'd sworn never to utter again in mixed company had escaped my lips without passing through the commonsense portion of my brain as I surveyed myself in the full-length, steam-covered bathroom mirror, my gaze focusing on what I believed to be my ever expanding midsection. Glancing up, Dave's eyes held mine for a brief second in the mirror before he nuzzled my neck with a quick kiss. Dropping his huge white towel momentarily, he embraced me by the offending midsection and pulled me closer. "You didn't answer me," I whispered, leaning my head back on his shoulder and still staring at the mirror. Dropping his arms from my waist Dave picked up the towel and quietly resumed caressing my back with the fluffy soft towel, moving slowly down my back following the curve of my spine to the natural division that separated the roundness of my behind; he seemed totally absorbed in what he was doing. "Dave," I whined softly, looking down at him on his knees as he gently stroked each of my legs, from top to bottom, while I stubbornly refused to let go of the question. Still quiet, Dave stood up, turned me toward the door, and gave me a playful slap on my bottom, sending me out of the bathroom. "I'm not going to answer you, because that's a trick question," he said, closing the bathroom door before I could register a complaint. I heard the hum of his electric razor, signaling the end of this conversation, as I sat naked and pouting on the bed. I wanted to be angry at Dave, but I was really angry at myself for exposing this pitiful part of my personality, and for knowing from previous conversations of this sort with this man that he was—dare I say it?—right. As much as I hate to admit it, that one question with those five little words "Do you think I'm fat?" had thrown me smack-dab in the middle of the comparison game, and Dave was refusing to play along with me. I really can't blame him for not answering, because he knew from previous experience that I can be difficult when it comes to areas in which I feel inadequate. For example, my inability to be fresh as a daisy the day after staying up all night to work.

"You seem a little tired and cranky; why don't you take a nap?"

"I'm not cranky, damn it! I know when I'm tired. Are we going to the movie or not?"

Or putting too much chili powder on his favorite Southwestern chicken because I wanted to surprise him by making it a little different.

"Honey, it's fine, honest, don't worry about it," he

rasped in a choking voice as he reached for his third glass of water. "I like my food spicy."

"You can't be serious. Your eyes started watering after the first bite." By now, Dave knew any answer he gave would only gain him the booby prize of my dissatisfaction: if he had said, "Yes, I think you're putting on a few pounds," I would have felt devastated. And if he had said, "No, I think you look just fine," I would have called his judgment into question. But I must say in all righteous self-defense that I was a ripe candidate for the fat question, due to my morning trip to the gym.

"Okay, people, lift those arms and stretch, now step left, step right, step up, step down, step one-two-three stretch, step left, step right, five more times, work those bodies, burn that fat!" the aerobic instructor yelled as she energetically bounced from side to side, swinging her arms high over her head. Situated in the back of the class I had a full view of the twenty women and three men moving in perfect unison like a well-oiled machine keeping up with the instructor, while I huffed and puffed trying to remember which was my right foot and which was my left. During our five-minute cooldown break, as I scanned the gym for an oxygen tank, or at the very least a phone so nobody would have to waste precious minutes screaming for one to call 911 when I passed out, I overheard a woman who was a dead ringer for Jada Pinkett tell another woman who I swear was Kate Moss's double that she wished the instructor would speed up the workout 'cause she was in a fat-burning mood and she wanted to look her sexy best tonight for a big date. While I consider my-

self somewhat of a workout buff, I usually move at my own pace. But after hearing several of my gym buddies tout the slimming virtues of aerobic workouts I had decided to give it a try, only to discover that I just don't really want to be that slim. Now as much as I profess to love all parts of myself, there are still times when I find myself falling into what seems to be that female-owned territory of physical self-deprecation.

Zoey, one of my best friends, says that physical dissatisfaction is linked to the X chromosome, thereby making it a female trait, and even in the absence of medical proof to the contrary, I'm inclined to believe her. Just the other day we were in the supermarket picking up a few things when I spotted the latest issue of one of my favorite women's magazines. I'm a magazine junkie by nature and every month come hell or high water I'm the first one at the local supermarket checkout counter, with my sometimes last few dollars, eager to buy my share of glossy-covered promises. Anyway, I was showing Zoey the cover, which happened to have a picture of a particularly beautiful Black model, and I remarked that I wished I looked that good. I mean this model had the kind of looks we all believe are too good to be real but that we try to imitate just the same. Zoey, in all of her infinite charm, rolled her eyes skyward (which should have been my first clue as to what was coming) and said, in a voice loud enough for the whole supermarket to hear:

"Sweetcakes, there ain't enough liposuction, make-up, or hair in the world to make you look like this here paper doll. In the first place she doesn't even look real and in the second place if the good Lord had'a wanted you to look like this woman you would've been her twin. Girl! I swear, you're just pitiful when it comes to all this tabloid madness. Now let's pay for all this stuff so I can get home—my ice cream's meltin'."

I have to admit tact has never been Zoey's strong point, but her addiction to reality is infectious at times. Like Dave, Zoey refuses to buy into the belief that beauty only comes in one flavor—youthful sexiness. I hate to admit it, it's not so much the magazine that sparks my interest as it is the model's image on the cover. While I generally feel good about myself most of the time, looking at that model in all of her perfection made me want to believe that I was somehow lacking in sexual attractiveness. When I looked at her perfectly shaped and made-up face, her perfect hair, and her very well-defined youthful body, how could I, standing in that checkout line wearing baggy jeans, no makeup, and a baseball cap, not find myself lacking in those areas? It's not that I want to be the model as much as I want to embody her youthful sexiness. In the real world I know that beauty and perfection don't equal sexiness, but in the perfect world of print media I'm seduced into believing that beauty, perfect body, and sex are somehow synonymous, and if I don't have the holy trinity or any one of the three I'm somehow lacking as a woman. I become irritated with myself for falling into the beauty comparison trap because I know it's false and generally based on someone else's perception of who and what will make me more appealing. But I also recognize how difficult it is for us everyday hit-the-ground-running women to teeter between the security of self-acceptance and the dark valley of self-doubt when we receive so many messages from the outside world that tell us that we're not okay in the looks department. Media messages like "To have beautiful, shining, sexy hair, use . . . ," "Build seductive abs in eight minutes," or "Boost your breasts without surgery" really feed into our sense of physical dissatisfaction and sexual attractiveness.

Recently a friend of mine complimented me on my discipline of going to the gym to work out five or six times a week. She told me that nothing short of Denzel Washington being her personal trainer could get her to work out on a regular basis. I wondered to myself what my friend would say if she ever saw me on one of my monthly binges of sitting naked, cross-legged in my overstuffed chair scarfing down a pint of butter pecan ice cream and reading articles entitled "50 Tips from Top Models on How to Enhance Your Personal Beauty." I tell myself that I'm working out for my health, but I also have to admit that the side benefit of hearing Dave tell me that I have a great body doesn't hurt either.

In my logical mind I know that beauty and sex aren't linked, but in my gut those two words fit together like hat and gloves, and I can't help wearing them from time to time. When I feel down about things happening in my life, I don't believe I'm beautiful or sexually attractive, and I'm more prone to asking "trick" questions in the hopes of boosting my vulnerable self-image. Dave knew that no matter how he answered my question I wouldn't be satisfied, because in reality it wasn't an issue about fat, it was more an issue of feeling physically vulnerable.

I know exactly what you're talkin' 'bout, sis. I've been strugglin' with my weight for years thinking that if I was thin I'd be more attractive. I've been on more diets than Carter's got liver pills, and I walk every day, but I'm still big. If one more person tells me I have a pretty face, but I'd really look good if I just lost a little weight I'll sit on them. I know I'm sexy 'cause I feel sexy and I've been married to Winyah for fifteen years so he must think I'm sexy too. To be real honest, sis, I'm a little surprised to hear you talk'n like this—after all, you're kind of the queen of self-esteem.

Roxy

What can I say, Roxy? Even us queens have our down days. I believe that I do have healthy self-esteem, but that doesn't mean that I'm immune to all the negative messages that we as women get on a daily basis. I'm starting to realize, thanks to Zoey's enlightened observation, that when I buy those magazines what I'm really buying is an image of glamour that exists in a world that doesn't really apply to my life. I've noticed that the majority of those cover models are in their twenties, an age I've long since passed. When I was twenty, I could match those models step for step, but I'm not twenty anymore and my body has gone through a number of natural life transitions. For instance, I'm still carrying some baby fat, you know, that pound or two that you gain during pregnancy—

and my baby's twenty-three years old. I've got what are modestly called laugh lines and wrinkles in places where I didn't even know I had places to get them. On my good days, when I'm at peace with myself, I take pride in my body, knowing that I've earned every pound, line, and wrinkle. But on those days when I've just bought out the supermarket magazine rack or I can't keep up with a rigorous gym workout I'm prone to devaluing my physical self. The people who publish those magazines aren't out to make me feel bad personally; they're doing their job, which is to sell a product. I know enough about myself to realize that I only start buying into what they're selling, youthful sexiness, when I'm feeling stressed in other areas of my life.

You know what's confusing for me is that being sexy doesn't have a thing to do with being beautiful, and beauty doesn't have anything to do with sex, yet when it comes to women those two things always seem to be put together. Now why is that?

Jonie

It's pretty much like I told sis—it's a gene thang.

Zoey

I believe it's more conditioning then anything else, Jonie. I think that as women we've been given messages that have led us to believe that beauty and sex are the only things we have to offer the world. Now like I said before, logically we know better—after all, women have been responsible for all types of world achievements. But when we pick up magazines, who do we see and read about—all the beautiful sexy women in the movie business. Just recently I read an article that not only gave the actress's weight but her dress size and all her beauty tips. Information like this makes it easy to get sucked in, especially when we're feeling vulnerable.

Honey, let me tell you something: you don't have to read magazines to feel vulnerable. The other night Philip and I were watching MTV with the boys and this video came on with these young girls made up to look twice their age, wearing these hot pants and tops small enough to fit in my change purse. Poor li'l Clay was in a trance he was starin' so hard, and my baby's only ten. Josh started doing all this yelling, about he really likes this song, when I told Phil to change the station. But it really made me mad watching these young girls shakin' and twistin' their behinds. I kept wondering to myself where in the world are their mothers, letting them do some trash like that.

Gracie

Let's face it—trashy sex sells. I bet that song is a million-dollar hit based on that one video. Actually I don't really have a problem with it as much as some folks do, but then again I don't have kids either. Shoot! When the mood strikes me, I'll throw on my hot pants, high heels, blond wig, and shake my moneymaker with the best of 'em. But at the same time I know that when I get up on Monday morning, put on my Donna Karan suit, and head for the office I'm still the same hot mama that I was on Saturday night. The only real difference is I know that Saturday is about hav'n fun and Monday is about business. A lot of young girls don't get to see the transition that a lot of these video stars make and they think that it's all about being out there sexually all the time.

Zoey

You know, I read an article recently in one of those business journals that said one of the quickest and surest ways to make money in the stock market is to invest in cosmetics companies or weight-management programs.

Stella

Girl, if that's true I better get me some 'cause we just started letting Kindra wear eye makeup and lipstick and she's the only person I know that can go through a whole tube of lipstick in a week. Leon looked at her this morning at breakfast and asked her what flavor she was this week. I swear that girl has enough eye shadow and lipstick in her bathroom to open up her own drugstore.

Cyree

My girl Summer is more into the natural look, so she isn't into the whole makeup thing, but last month she decided that she wants to wear dreads so she went to the hairdresser and got her hair all parted and twisted to start them growing. I know they'll look good when they grow out, but she keeps her head covered in a scarf and I ain't seen my baby's head in so long till I forget what it looks like.

Queenie

You know I wasn't too worried about it but maybe I should be paying a little more attention, because Arletta has been making noises about going on a diet because she's too fat. She wants to start taking dance lessons in the fall, and she keeps talking about getting in shape. Now you all have seen Arletta and she don't weigh a hundred pounds soakin' wet. I've just been tossing it off and telling her not to worry about her weight, but maybe I better start watching her, 'cause she's only twelve and I don't want her developing any eating disorders.

Jonie

I think that would be a good idea, Jonie. If we as adults can get sucked into the whole beauty-is-thinness sexual trap, it's twice as easy for our daughters and younger sisters to get caught up in it.

Shoot! I was almost thirty years old before I started wearing makeup, and eatin' was always a main event in our house so I never even heard the word "diet" till I got to college. Now we got to worry about all this stuff not only for ourselves, but for our kids as well.

Gracie

Child, this reminds me of the time I fell over a pair of my shoes and almost broke my neck trying to back out of a room in the dark. It was the first time me and Willie had gone to bed together, and I had to use the bathroom—well, I didn't want him to see my big be-hind, so I thought I'd be cute and leave the lights off and back out of the room. Well, honey, one minute I was on my feet and the next I was clutching air. I was so 'shamed, when I told Willie why I was backin' out of the room, he said, "Woman, you must be out of your mind. Why you think I'm wit' you? I like my woman with a bit of meat on her; it just means there's more to love." We been together ever since. I guess I'm just lucky that Summer don't seem to have any hang-ups about her body, 'cause she's big in places just like me, but she's a pretty girl, and I make sure I tell her she's pretty 'cause I don't want her depending on no man having to tell her.

Queenie

I'm glad your validating Summer's attractiveness early, Queenie. I think being attractive is more a sense of feeling than it is a sense of actually being. Giving our daughters and sons messages about their physical attractiveness allows them to start having a sense of self-worth early, making them less vulnerable to someone else's opinion of who and how they should be as a person.

Well, I don't care what nobody says. I know what helps me feel and look my best, and if they ain't got

Flori Roberts cosmetics in heaven I won't be making a personal appearance.

> *Zoey*

Zoey, girl sometimes you so scandalous it's a shame.

> *Roxy*

Why, I ain't tellin' no lie, I'm into personal physical enhancement and cosmetics do it for me. Sis just said feeling good about yourself is what makes you attractive and I believe her. Wearing makeup helps me feel attractive.

> *Zoey*

I think you make a good point, Zoey, just as long as you know you're doing it for yourself and not because somebody else wants you to wear the makeup. Let's face it, physical self-enhancement isn't a bad thing, but it can become negative if we do it for the wrong reasons, and in my book all the wrong reasons start with so-and-so doesn't like the way my hair, body, skin, nose, or whatever looks, so maybe I'd better change it. If we choose to change something based on our own sense of need or want that's different. That's why Dave didn't answer when I asked the fat question—he knew that it had to be my decision to make whatever changes I was going to make. He was attracted to the woman he met, not to the woman he felt I needed to become. Looking at my relationship with Dave helps me to realize just how far I've come in terms of self-acceptance, especially when I think about my first sexual experience.

I was twenty-one, living on my own for the first time with two college roommates in our very own apartment. I met Dave on a blind date when one of my roommates fixed me up with her boyfriend's best friend. I knew I liked him on our first date. He was tall, handsome, and had a great sense of humor. He was in the service, had been married and was now divorced, and had traveled quite a bit, which made him seem worldly and wise to my young college-girl eyes. We had several dates and after spending one beautiful Saturday afternoon on the beach, where I wore my cutest short set and laughed at every word that escaped his sugar-coated lips, we returned to the apartment to find ourselves alone, and one kiss led to another and another led to more passion, which led to the bedroom.

"How was I?" I asked with some anxiety after we'd made love.

"You were wonderful. Now go to sleep."

"Are you sure?"

"Yes, now go to sleep."

"Do you love me?"

"Yes, baby, I do. Now will you please let me get some sleep?"

Since it was my first partnered sexual experience, I was naive and needed reassurance. I was scared and wanted to talk about things—mainly the thing that had just occurred. I read and interpreted his tired state as indifference, disinterest, and my not being "good enough." So while he slept, I had the entire night to think, or should I say worry, about all the "important stuff." Stuff like, did I do it right? Was I too fat? Were my breasts too small? But most of all, was he pleased with me? . . . Oh God! what if I was pregnant? Would he marry me? . . . It didn't matter that he told me he was pleased. After all, he only told me after I had asked and we all know that doesn't count. I hated having questions and not having answers, not that I would have believed him 'cause I had heard guys talk about girls they'd slept with and I knew the score. How would I know if I had really pleased him? What were the signs? Who could I trust to give me the information I needed? I needed to talk to somebody, but who? Maybe I could call Momi; she'd understand—or would she? I found myself grappling with these questions at two o'clock in the morning cuddled next to Rip Van Winkle after what seemed like hours of passionate lovemaking. I wanted to talk, and my roommates seemed like a logical choice, so I slipped carefully out of bed and crept to their bedrooms, but to my surprise neither one of them was home. I went into the living room and lay on the couch to think, and spotting the phone in the kitchen I contemplated for what seemed like the hundredth time calling my mother.

As I mentally calculated the time difference between California and New Jersey, not wanting to frighten her by calling too early (Momi wasn't at her best in the early morning), I thought about what I would say. Hi, Momi, I'm okay but I just had sex for the first time and what I want to know is . . . I fell asleep before I could make the call, thinking about all the questions I wanted to ask my mother. I knew my mother well enough to know that had I actually made that call she would have fussed at me for being "so fast," even at my ripe age of twenty-one, but she would have had the patience to listen to my concerns. As I was growing up, from time to time we had discussed the general topic of being in love but the finer details of carnal lust just never entered the conversation. I got the general "You'll know when it's right" kind of answer whenever I inquired about love, and because I believed everything Momi told me at that time in my life, I believed that I would know when it was right. But I was wrong; I didn't know, and I was scared about not knowing. I eventually discovered what I needed to know about love and sex, in pretty much the same way we all manage to learn new things, on my own through trial and error. Some of the trial was sweet, passionate, and even laughable, but the error was often filled with hurt and disappointment. Dave was sensitive enough to recognize that I had the key to my "trick question" and with time I would give myself the answer.

Dear Journal,

It's been a week since I let the fat question slip through my lips, and I've since had some time to talk with my sister friends about the merits of physical self-acceptance in this world based on youthful beauty and sexiness. When I looked in my mirror this evening I saw my mother's face and body staring back at me when she was about my age. My relatives tell me how much I favor her, and I've always denied the resemblance, wanting to create and define my own image. I wanted to be my own woman from bottom to top, in appearance and thought. I made the mistake of believing that if I looked like her, I would become who she was, a woman who because of her ethnicity didn't fit into a social system that refused to value her beauty as a Black woman in her own right. I wanted to challenge that system, proving once and for all that beauty doesn't have to conform to culturally defined standards. The woman I saw tonight in my mirror—smooth, honey-colored skin, copper-colored hair, bright eyes with just a hint of mischief, a mouth born for laughter and sass, full bosom, rounded firm stomach, standing tall on strong, well-shaped legs—was not only me; it was Momi too—even I couldn't dispute this reality. My mother was physically beautiful, and I look like her. I may forget that from time to time; but when I forget in my stressed-out tabloid madness, "am I fat?" trick question, physically vulnerable down times, all I have to do is look in the mirror. Momi will be standing right there ready to remind me of just how beautiful and sexy I really am.

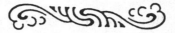

PLAYING WITH FIRE

I learned the art of flirting from my mother. Of course she would never in a million years admit to this little-known fact. But what else do you call it when someone's eyes dance with sweet mischief, her laughter rings with playfulness, and there's just enough sass in each word to make her invitingly spicy? Momi had all of these qualities plus more, and she was one of the prettiest women I'd ever seen. In all honesty flirting is not an activity with which Momi would ever have identified. It was something she associated with being a hussy, as in "look'a how she's act'n, she ain't nothing but a hussy." If the "she" in question was really outrageous in her behavior the descriptive adjective "shameless" was added for extra measure. Generally "she" who found herself singled out in such a fashion was doing nothing more than enjoying the attention that men were willing to bestow on her. From my limited vantage point as an observant teenager, it appeared that the behaviors (outside of being noticed by men, that is) that most often seemed to get women labeled "hussy" by Momi and her friends were quite innocent: smiling shyly, being quietly pretty, appearing helpless, or, on the other hand, being confident in the company of more than one man at a time (otherwise known as "holding court") and seeking out the company of men when other women were present. Being a "shameless hussy" took a little more work: dressing provocatively in order to attract attention, feeling confident enough to think you were cute even if others didn't think so, switching or swinging your hips, batting your eyes, being bold enough to obviously seek out the attention of men, coyly speaking your mind in mixed company by adding just the right amount of humor or sass to your words, holding court and being loud about it, and the real biggie, flirting openly with a married man or a man who you knew to be in a "committed relationship." Young girls who behaved in such a manner were considered "fast," while women over twenty-one who behaved in a similar fashion were considered "shameless hussies." For whatever reasons, and to this day I'm not clear why it is, attractive women who enjoyed the attention of men were and still are considered (by some of us) to be phony or "put on," as Momi would say. Momi was neither fast nor a hussy, nor was her behavior a put-on—but she was, in fact, a flirt by nature. Her flashing gray eyes, inviting laughter, and sassy temperament were as natural as her honey-colored skin and copper-colored hair. Men, women, and children were drawn to her because she was a delightful, charming, funny woman who loved to laugh. My mother was also a romantic woman who loved pretty clothes, flowers, and the sense of order that she gave to everything within her reach. It's easy to see why my father was attracted to and loved her. My parents were married for fifty-three years, and while they had their ups and downs they were for the most part a very romantic couple; up until the day she died I never heard my father call her anything but honey.

In all fairness I have to say that everything I ever learned about how to attract a man I learned from my mother. I use to love studying her behavior as she playfully flirted with Daddy across the dinner table, or sat in his lap when they watched television together. When Momi wanted Daddy's attention she got it. And for all her playfulness and love she didn't "take no stuff" as she liked to say, because when she had something to say you can believe she didn't bite her tongue. Being the oldest girl, and having had the longest opportunity to observe her behavior while I was growing up, I share many of my mother's traits, some more than others, but the trait of hers that I loved and imitated the most (and the one that she cared for the least in me) was the art of flirting. It was tough having a role model that didn't want you to model her behavior, but somehow I managed to learn how to attract the attention of men without becoming a hussy in my mother's eyes. However, I must admit she always did consider me "fast," much to her obvious dismay.

Some experts in the field of psychology say that mothers very often feel threatened as their daughters approach womanhood. It's my theory that mothers aren't so much threatened as they are fearful. I believe that mothers instinctively fear that their daughters will become victims of circumstances that can lock them into hard lifetime situations. In my case, it wasn't my fast behavior that disturbed my mother as much as it was what the flirting implied—my impending sexuality. My flirtatious behavior at age sixteen signaled to my mother that I had some knowledge of who I was as a woman and the power that awareness gave me.

Because my mother had only her own limited experience to draw from, she viewed my so-called fast behavior as dangerous. I was continually being made aware of my behavior, especially around boys. I have numerous memories of being told to be a "good girl" or to "watch myself" so as not to get in trouble, but no one ever said the word *sex*. Momi assumed that I knew, but never said, and I thought I knew, but never asked, who I was being good for and what kind of trouble I was supposed to stay out of. I also believe that my mother, like other mothers of her era, knew that she could warn me of the dangers, but she couldn't stop me from becoming a sexual woman, and felt helpless in the process. As my mother viewed it, my flirtatious behavior equaled sexual behavior and confirmed her sense of helplessness because she didn't know how to tell me to set limits. In my mother's world (which was dictated by her upbringing and the church) there were two kinds of women who had sex: good women, i.e., women who were married, and bad women who weren't married. She took her role as mother very seriously when it came to raising her daughters to be "good women."

"My dream is for you to grow up, go to college, and settle down with some nice young man to raise a family," Momi would often lecture whenever I moaned and groaned about not having a steady boyfriend. Actually I felt like Momi and I were reading the same book, but she was just on a different page. I wanted the very same things that she wanted for me; it's just that I wanted to start with the boyfriend sooner rather than later.

Actually I enjoy the art of flirting. Mainly, my enjoyment comes from feeling attractive and wanting to share my sense of attractiveness with others. In fact, I can honestly say that flirting has kept me out of more trouble than it's gotten me into, because when I feel attractive there's less chance that I will choose to seek out confirmation from someone else. My mother was fearful that flirting would lead me into sexual temptation, and as an adult I can't deny that at times the innocent behavior of "being fast" did result in some interesting outcomes, but that was my choice, not a direct result. I truly believe that flirting can be a sense of self-confirmation that appears when a woman knows who she is inwardly and feels secure enough to show the world that playful side of herself.

Well, I may be outta line here but I agree with your mother, flirting don't lead to nothing but trouble for young girls. They're already fast enough. We've got babies out there now having babies, and flirting with all these little hot-tailed boys only speeds up the process.

Queenie

49

The last time I checked, Queenie, the only thing that led to young women having babies was sex with young men. Flirting doesn't necessarily lead to sex; it can but it doesn't have to, especially when people observe the proper boundaries. If we start schooling our daughters and younger sisters early about setting proper limits, we won't have to worry about them going buck wild with every little boy they meet.

Zoey

I agree with Zoey on this one, Queenie. Flirting isn't dangerous when we know our own personal limits. True, some flirtatious behaviors can go from innocent to dangerous in a heartbeat, but for the most part it's pretty harmless. We have to give our younger sisters the word that it's okay to feel and express their sense of personal attractiveness; however, some of their signals of attractiveness may be misinterpreted as signs of sexual readiness and it's always appropriate to say "no" when they find themselves in that situation. I think part of our problem is that we're doing to our daughters and younger sisters the same thing that our mothers did to us—believing that flirting can and only does lead to being sexual. We have to be willing to tell them about setting limits, by giving permission to say no and trusting them to do the right thing. Personally I believe that our younger sisters are making mistakes because as adults we're not giving them proper information.

Seems to me with all this information they got out here nowadays they don't need for us to tell them nothin'.

Queenie

There is a lot of information on sex out there, Queenie, but younger sisters still need to hear from us too.

Sis, you and Zoey kept using the words "boundaries" and "limits"—just what kind of personal boundaries and limits are you talking about here?

Stella

Take it, sis.

Zoey

Thanks, Zoey. Woman to woman, my flirtatious behavior would be different because my intent would be different. As for myself, when I'm attracted to someone I don't know, I show initial interest by smiling, making eye contact, and if I really feel bold I'll strike up an innocent conversation to get a sense of who he is and to see if there's a response. If I find that I want to know him better and if his response is favorable we may set aside some time to get better acquainted. I've actually met a number of interesting people this way and these situations haven't all led to me having sex with the person. When I'm interested in a sexual connection I turn up the heat on my advances but if I discover—usually after our first conversation—that I'm not interested in going any further I just let the contact die a natural death.

I'm more the shameless hussy type myself. To me flirting is about making a sexual connection and I know that going into the game. I don't flirt to make friends, I flirt when I feel a certain sexual attraction toward someone. I'm like sis in that I believe in testing the waters first with some conversation to see if the feeling's mutual. If it is I make my intentions known; if it isn't I move on about my business. If I'm not interested in you after that first conversation, then like sis, I just let it go.

Zoey

Damn, Zoey, that sounds so cold and calculated. Don't you believe in love, girl?

Gracie

Sure I believe in love. You all believe it's calculated and cold because I know what I want my end result to be and I'm going after it. I think love and romance is nice in its proper place. I've been there and had that and make no mistake, when I'm ready I'll have it again. But I don't happen to think that having sex just for the fun of it is wrong as long as I'm careful. Sis and I use pretty much the same methods. It's just that we want different endings: sis flirts with possibilities in mind; I do it with action in mind.

Zoey

I don't think sex is wrong, I just think it needs to happen between adult people who really care about each other. I don't want my child to grow up flirting from one man to the next just to have a good time with sex. I want her to find somebody she can love, respect, and maybe someday marry. Her body is much too precious to be giving it to every Tom, Dick, and Harry she may think she likes. If that's what flirting will get her then I want her to leave it the hell alone.

Stella

I think we have to remember that flirting and sex are two separate acts. I believe that flirting is kind of safe because it's generally a fairly public act, whereas sex is private. I don't know about Zoey, but my experiences with flirting have rarely gone from batting my eyes at somebody one minute to jumping in bed with him in the next minute.

My experiences haven't been minute to minute like that either. Now it may happen that I'll meet somebody early in the evening and we end up spending the night together, but that's only if I want it to happen that way.

Zoey

Child! I'm sitting over here stressin' just listening to this conversation. Just the mere thought of someone other than me seeing my twelve-year-old baby without her clothes on, even when she's an adult, makes me break out in a cold sweat. She's already talking about how cute some li'l boy is that goes to her school, and I'll be real honest, I ain't even ready to go there yet. Right about now I just want to lock her in a closet till she turns twenty-one. Lord, honey, if I feel this way and she's only twelve I'll probably have a nervous breakdown by the time she reaches sixteen.

Jonie

I know how you feel, Jonie, 'cause I felt that same way about Summer, but she's seventeen and I just have to thank the good Lord every night for helping her keep her head. I ain't gonna lie, I've done my share of flirting, harmless and shameless. I've been on both sides of the track, but I don't want Summer to follow in my footsteps, and so far as I know she hasn't. I thank God every day for Willie, 'cause who knows where me and my child would have ended up or who we would have ended up with if he hadn't come into my life when he did. Being with Willie really helped me turn my life around; he ain't no saint but he sure helped me avoid living a life of sin. Now I don't expect Summer to be no angel either, but I do expect her to use her head where men are concerned.

Queenie

You know, Jonie, I think I know why you and Stella get nervous. I think we all get nervous when it comes to thinking about our kids being sexual. I think we get nervous because it's like Queenie said, at one time or another we've all been on both sides of the flirting track—I know I have—and it can be scary, but it doesn't have to be that way if we make it our business to talk to our kids about sex before they become curious about it on their own. It's like I was telling Queenie before, there's plenty of information out there for our kids, but they need to hear from us too. We've got to be willing to break the code of fear that our mothers gave us when it comes to talking about sex and give our kids some direct solid information.

Okay, sis, you just lost me—what code of fear are you talking about?

Cyree

Well, remember when I told you that we never talked about sex in my house when I was in my teens? Momi couldn't bring herself to talk openly to me about sex because I believe she didn't have the language, so she would code her message in saying things like "I want you to be good," or if she saw me flirting, she'd say, "Don't be so fast, miss, you'll be grown soon enough." Then there were the lectures when I was in high school, "Keep your head in the books and leave those li'l boys alone." When I started dating I heard, "I want you to come back in this house the same way you left" or "Don't think you're going to start dating, and bringing trouble home to my doorstep, so you just watch yourself."

Well, I don't hear that your mother told you anything wrong or bad, so what's the problem? You knew what she was talkin' about. She just didn't want you to get in any trouble and frankly that makes plenty sense to me.

Queenie

You're right, Queenie. My mother didn't tell me anything bad, and I did understand her messages when I got older, but the implied message was one of distrust. There was also the undertone in my mother's messages that feeling sexual was somehow wrong or bad,

55

and I believed as I got older that if I had those types of feelings then there must be something wrong or bad about me too. In reality, as we mature, starting in adolescence, we all, girls and boys, experience certain attractions that could be considered sexual feelings. Our kids may not interpret those feelings as sexual, so we might hear them say something like "I really like so-and-so" or "I have a crush on so-and-so." Then we start doing what our mothers did with us—we give them our fears about being sexual. I think we're really playing with fire if we don't give our younger sisters and brothers honest messages.

> *I'm there with you, sis. I've already started schoolin'*
> *Kindra about the facts of life. We've had some really*
> *good talks and now that she's sixteen and she's*
> *started dating I want her to know how she can take*
> *care of herself.*
>
> *Cyree*

I'm curious, Cyree. What did you tell Kindra?

> *I was pretty up-front with her. I told her that she's a*
> *beautiful and intelligent young woman and young*
> *men are going to be attracted to her and she is going*
> *to be attracted to them too. I told her that being at-*
> *tracted and having feelings are natural, but just be-*
> *cause she felt a certain way it didn't mean that she*
> *had to act on the feelings. But if there was ever a time*
> *when she felt confused or pressured she should excuse*
> *herself and call me so that we could talk. And honey,*

I promptly went out and bought her a cell phone just to make sure she had something to call me on.

Cyree

Come on, Cyree, be real—what's the chance that Kindra's gonna call you in the heat of the moment?

Nonie

Honey, she can call the woman in the moon for all I care as long as she does something to give herself a chance to think about the situation. Actually, I'm not too worried about Kindra because she has a good head on her shoulders, and I have enough faith to believe that she'll do the right thing.

Cyree

I like it that you thought of a way to give Kindra options and at the same time you helped her to feel good about herself.

Leon and I have been teachers for too many years and we've watched how these young kids act toward each other—they start talking about going steady in the third grade and by the time they're in the tenth grade they're parents. It's a sin and a shame the way some of these kids start messing up their lives before they've had a chance to really experience life. Leon and I talked early on about how we would approach the subject of sex with our kids. I didn't want to raise our daughter the way I was raised, ashamed of my body, never thinking I was attractive. And Leon said he didn't want Leon Jr. and James to think that they could use women like Kleenex, so he agreed to talk to the boys and I would talk to Kindra. Leon Jr. is four-teen so he'll be out there dating soon and James is only ten but it's better to start early than to wait till it's too late.

Cyree

Well, I may be old-fashioned, but I told Summer the same thing that my mother told me: make sure you come back the same way you left. And it must have worked 'cause she's been good so far, and if she hasn't I don't want to know about it. I told Summer a long time ago that a lot of these boys are only after one thing and she knows they'll tell a girl anything she wants to hear just to get it. But like I said, my baby seems to have her head on straight.

Queenie

What if Summer is gay?

Nonie

Don't go startin' no mess, Nonie. Why you always want to play with my head?

Queenie

I ain't startin' no mess. I just asked, that's all. I mean, it's a valid question. My mother told me the same thing your mother told you, and I always came back

58

the same way I left, mainly because I was messing with women. She told me to be careful of boys, not girls, and I was careful with boys, but I was attracted to girls. She never asked, and I never told her. I'm just wondering if the same rules would apply if she were attracted to women instead of men.

Nonie

Well, I know my child and I know she's attracted to men. Willie and I raised her in a solid Christian home, and I just know she doesn't think like that. If she felt that way I would know it by now. Summer's pretty open about most things.

Queenie

You might want to watch yourself there, sister woman, 'cause some of the most sincere Christians I know are gay and lesbian. Besides, the last time I checked religion didn't have a thing to do with a person's sexual orientation. Sex is sex and religion is religion—that's where the similarities begin and end.

Zoey

I'm not saying that being gay is wrong or nothing; all I'm saying is I just know my child, and either way I don't want to know about it. Sex is private far as I'm concerned and who you do it with is your own business. I just want Summer to make good choices and to have a sense of dignity and respect for herself.

Queenie

You know, Queenie, I can respect where you're coming from when you talk about having dignity and respect for one's self. I would also agree that Nonie's question is valid—do the messages about sex change if our children's sexual orientation is different? Personally I think my message to my son would be the same, who you choose to have sex with is your choice, but whoever you choose, just make sure you use protection, because there are sexual risks and personal responsibilities for gays and lesbians too, and your life will depend on your decisions about safety.

You know I've often wondered how I would take it if one of my boys told me he was gay. At any rate I know I'd take it better than Phil would—that man's so homophobic it's a shame. But I would want to know, because I don't ever want my kids to feel they can't talk to me about anything and that includes who they're in love with in their lives.

Gracie

I can't honestly say how I would react, because I don't have kids. My niece Toni is lesbian and she's been out for years and she brings her girlfriend over whenever they come to visit from California, and it's no big deal. Winyah is pretty open-minded; I guess it's because he works with all those street kids. But I do think we have to start talking to all our kids about sex.

Roxy

You know I wanted to tell my mother how I felt about loving women a long time ago, but I just knew she wouldn't hear me. She felt the same way you do, Queenie; I guess that's why I never said anything, but I would have loved to talk to her about it. I think not being able to talk openly with her is one of the reasons that I made so many mistakes along the way to getting where I am in life. I did a lot of pretending. I pretended to like boys and I even got married just to please her, and I have to admit it was because I was confused too, not about who or what I wanted but mainly because I didn't know what to do about it . . . the "it" being sex. In that whole process of getting married two people got hurt, me and the man I married. Frank and I are on pretty good terms today, but I'm just sorry we had to go through all that.

Nonie

Who did you talk to, Nonie?

Stella

This may surprise you, but it was my grandmother. Nana, my father's mother. When I told her how I felt about LaShay, after my divorce from Frank, Nana told me she'd suspected that I was gay for a long time but never said anything because she didn't want to put any ideas in my head if they weren't already there. I think Nana told Daddy, and Daddy told my mother. Daddy's pretty cool about my relationship with La-Shay, but Mom still blames LaShay because she thinks Shay broke up my marriage. I tried to tell her in a hundred different ways that it's not LaShay's fault but she just doesn't want to hear it. But I'll always love my Nana for hearing what my mother can't accept.

Nonie

You know as much as this conversation is scaring the life out of me, I know I'm gonna have to tell Arletta the facts of life at some point. I don't want my child to be scared of sex, I want her to enjoy it and be comfortable with herself in any situation. I can remember my mother always told me that if I ever got in a situation where my feelings got the better of my mind, that I should remember to hear her voice telling me to take a deep breath, just take a deep breath, baby. Mama told me that when I was fourteen, and she's been gone for ten years now and I can still hear her telling me to just take a deep breath whenever I'm in a tight spot. My sister's daughter Connie just turned seventeen and the other day she asked me to take her to Planned Parenthood because she wants to get some birth control pills. I asked her if she'd done anything, you know, been with a boy, and she told me no, and I believe her. Honey, I did some real heavy breathing on that one, and I told her that I wanted her to talk to her mom first, and if her mom wouldn't go with her then I would go. I know DeeDee, my sister, will hit the ceiling because she still thinks Connie is a little kid, and besides, she doesn't think kids Connie's age should be thinking about sex, but I've told her time and time again that Connie's at an age where she's gonna be interested in boys and she needs to talk to her. But DeeDee's like me in some ways I guess—we can't imagine our kids growing up. If DeeDee won't go with Connie then I will 'cause my niece is a good kid and I don't want to see her get messed up. But you know what I'm gonna tell her and Arletta when she's old enough, just what mama told me: take a deep breath, baby, just take a deep breath before you do anything.

Jonie

Well, baby, as scared as you might be, we really got to talk to our kids. Just the other day I overheard one of Renee's friends telling her she wasn't worried about her man coming back to her 'cause she knew she was his "number one bitch." Now this young girl is Renee's age, eighteen, all right, and she's got a baby by this joker who's out in the streets doing only God knows what with who, and she's talking about being his number one bitch. I don't like the idea that Renee keeps hanging with her, but I've tried to stay out of the way of her picking her friends. Anyway, after she left I asked Renee what was up with this number one bitch business, and Renee just says, "Ah, don't sweat it, Mom"; Tootie—that's her friend—just means that she's still Donta's main girlfriend, 'cause she's got his baby. Well, I told Renee that I hope she wasn't looking to be no guy's number one girlfriend in that kind of way, 'cause if she was she could just pack her bags right now 'cause her father and I ain't havin' it. Honey, Renee looked at me like I was crazy, 'cause I'm sure I sounded like I was, and told me, "Mommy, you know you and Daddy raised me with more sense than *that. I ain't looking to have anybody's baby or anything else till I'm at least thirty-five. I got too much I want to do with my life." Child, you don't know how happy I was to hear those words come out of her mouth. Peer pressure is so strong nowadays till you just have to watch everything these kids do. I may be naive in thinking my child hasn't messed around at some point, but at least from all indications that I've seen and heard she's being safe. Frankly, with all this information about AIDS and STDs going around I'm surprised when I hear about any girl getting pregnant nowadays. If I was single again I wouldn't even want to know what a naked penis looked like. Shoot, the way some of these folks from social service agencies have been standing on street corners passing them out, I'm beginning to think that condoms are the only thing a person can get for free these days.*

Stella

I know what you're saying, Stella; even with all the information available on sexually transmitted diseases and AIDS, some of us, young and old alike, are still willing to take unnecessary risks in the sexual intercourse department. I just read some information stating that there continues to be an increase in the number of teenagers and women of color who are contracting and dying from STDs and AIDS and that really scares me. I'm just glad that we're all willing to talk to our kids about being safe. I have to admit it is frightening to know that some of our younger sisters are so willing to settle for less than they actually deserve when it comes to giving up their self-respect and dignity in order to be with someone who doesn't value them.

That's what I've been saying all long. Telling our kids that it's okay to flirt is like giving them permission to do other things. Sometimes I just think we give our kids too much information. I'm just glad I started raising Summer in the church.

Queenie

Listen up, sweetcakes, 'cause I thought we covered this ground about sex and religion. There's a whole lot of young church sisters out there pushin' baby strollers nowadays and the Lord didn't have a thing to do with it.

Zoey

Hold up, Zoey. I understand where Queenie's coming from—she needs to believe that there's a solid answer or solution to keeping her daughter safe. You know, Queenie, I really wish the church could provide us with the divine protection that we need and want, but it just doesn't work that way. It's true our religious beliefs provide us with a moral structure. But we can't make the mistake of believing that that structure is by any means shelter, especially when it comes to feeling sexual and predicting human behavior. After all, most of us were raised with some form of religion, but it's like Zoey said, in the heat of passion few if any of us think to call on the Lord.

Honey, I know that's right 'cause, I don't know about anybody else in here, the last time I called on the Lord in bed religion didn't have a thing to do with it.

Zoey

Zoey! You oughta be shame. I'm gonna pray overtime for you 'cause, girl, at the rate you're goin' you're gonna go straight to hell sure as I'm sittin' here. But I still believe we tell our kids too much.

Queenie

Thanks for your prayers, Queenie. I'll remember you in mine too.

Zoey

I don't think anybody can ever have too much information. Most of the kids that find themselves in trouble are the ones that don't have information. Let's be real—at some point we all need and want some outside validation concerning our sense of personal sexual attractiveness. We've got to face the facts, and the main fact is, our kids are going to make the decision to be sexual, just like we all made that decision for ourselves. I want my child, and yours too, to make an informed decision based on valid real information, not stuff they've picked up in the streets. We can't be stingy with sexual information; if we know it we've got an obligation to share what we know with them. Our kids trust us to tell them the truth and I believe they get pissed off when we don't share that truth with them up front. Personally I can't think of anything that I'd rather share more than information that will help them to be sexually safe, especially if that information helps them to make a better choice in their own life.

How do we know they're even listening to us? Besides, sis, you got it easy—you've got a son and you don't have to worry about him coming home pregnant.

Stella

I don't know that I have it any easier then anybody else, Stella. You're right, I don't have to worry about him coming home pregnant. I have to worry about him exposing himself to STDs, by having sex with a prostitute or drug user. That he might be in a sexually experimental stage or be gay and have unprotected sex with a man and be more at risk of getting AIDS. I've had to tell my son the same things you're telling your daughters, along with the message that having sexual intercourse is an adult decision that requires adult responsibilities. I had to tell him that having un-protected sex with a young woman could mean that she might end up pregnant and she will have to carry any irresponsible decision he makes for nine months and he'll have to support it for eighteen years and maybe more. And then I asked him if he was ready for that type of commitment. My son is real aware of what it's like to be raised by a single parent; I'm sure that lesson wasn't lost on him. And like the rest of us here with kids, I'm proud of the fact that he shares my values when it comes to children and their care. When he was younger, I used to take him with me whenever I volunteered at Planned Parenthood, so I've always talked to him about the need to be safe sexually for himself and for the safety of others in his life. As far as how do we know if our kids are listening, well, all I've got to say is we don't really know if they are unless they show us by their actions. And from what I've heard you all say, it sounds as if your kids heard your messages loud and clear. They may choose not to acknowledge your words at some point down the road, but at least all of our kids know that we're open to listening if they need or want to talk.

You know, I've just been sittin' here trippin' on that whole church thing because it's really bothering me. Queenie, you may not know this but I got put out of my church when I got pregnant with Arletta. Well, I didn't exactly get put out, but I was made to feel so shame and uncomfortable till I left. I used to be in the choir, and Mama was one of the mothers of the church and everything. Our whole family had been goin' to that church for years, but the minute I got pregnant everything changed. I got put out of the choir, and the reverend's wife called Mama and told her that it was a shame and disgrace that her and Daddy let me get myself in trouble. Mama was so hurt, and I thought Daddy was gonna have a fit. I did what I did on my own; Mama and Daddy didn't have nothing to do with it. That's what hurt me the most. We ended up joining another church, but that one experience put me off religion for a long time. Mainly the reason I went back was because Mama said that it wasn't right not to bring Arletta up in a church home. But I just had to say that 'cause sis is right; I was raised in the church and I still tested the waters so to speak.

Jonie

I'm glad you didn't give up on your religion, Jonie, and I'm really sorry that you and your family were treated badly by those who represented the church. But I guess we have to look at the facts and say that most religious institutions, including our own, have a real double standard when it comes to women's sexuality. A number of churches have some beliefs concerning our sexual behaviors. Personally I don't believe it's the churches' beliefs as much as it is the people's belief that head the churches. My former religious home frowned on divorce and sex outside of marriage. At first I felt really angry, hurt, and lost, but like you, Jonie, I found another means of being close to God.

Well, I consider myself to be a good Christian woman, and I've been divorced twice. I'm like you sis, I don't think it's the church that makes it hard but I do believe that some of the folks running the church get a little carried away. I went and talked to Pastor Mark when Phil and I first got together, and he told me that as long as I used good judgment it was my call, not his. I really respected him for that.

Gracie

Well that's what you'd find at my church, Gracie. As rocky as my past has been, I didn't think I would ever have a church home. But Reverend Honeywell and the whole congregation opened their arms in welcome to me, Summer, and Willie.

Queenie

You and Gracie are really fortunate to belong to a church and have pastors that are so open and accepting. I've heard horror stories from some single and divorced sisters about their experiences with the church.

Yeah, and I'm one of them. I've been told so many times that I'm going to hell because of my sexual orientation until I've given up countin'. I've heard it from my family, from the church, and from the community. You would think that after all this time folks would wake up and smell the coffee. Mama was big on preaching that God made us all and loves us all equally, and I believed her. But when she found out I was a lesbian, she dropped that speech and me real quick. LaShay was raised Catholic and she grew up believing everything was a sin, so she just left the church altogether. I found a nice church in the University District and I've been going over there but LaShay says thanks but no thanks.

Nonie

After I left my church home I found a lot of comfort in being spiritual. I find it more comforting to accept and be with God in a much more inclusive way. I can choose to attend any type church services if I want fellowship, but I know that even if I don't attend or belong to a church God will always be a part of my life.

Sis, you've mentioned this spiritual thing before. Just what is it anyway?

Roxy

For me, Roxy, spirituality is more a way of being. Let me see if I can put it into words. I believe in the basic goodness of all humankind because I believe that God resides in all of us. In many ways spirituality resembles many religions but without the dogma and rigid confines of believing that there's only one way to worship or speak with God. In a sense, I think of spirituality as all the good stuff from every possible religion rolled into one. Personally, I think that all forms of religion have something to offer, but it makes me uncomfortable when religion and churches dictate a person's lifestyle, especially when it comes to consenting adults. In my mind and heart God is all-accepting.

I'm with you on that one, sis, 'cause the God I believe in believes in sex too, and doesn't hand out rejection slips when you do the heathen thing every once in a while.

Zoey

Lord please help her.

Queenie

71

As I sat talking and listening to my sister friends share the various ways in which they were coping with the idea of their children being sexual and our own struggles with sex and religion it became clear to me that many of the struggles that our mothers had had still existed for us in some ways. Is flirting really dangerous? Does it always lead to sex? Should we talk to our kids about sex or shouldn't we? How do we tell them? What do we tell them and when? Do we need to know when they decide to be sexually active, or is it better not to know? Does the message remain the same if my child's sexual orientation is different? How do we give our kids options? Can we still embrace God if we choose to be sexual outside of marriage? Will God embrace us? I'm sure our mothers struggled with many of these same questions, but the major difference is we were struggling together out loud, exchanging ideas, thoughts, and opinions, talking in realistic language (not in codes, as our mothers had done), holding our fears up to the light. We weren't all in agreement and we didn't have all the answers, but we were talking. In listening to our conversation as sister friends I wondered what would have been different if my mother had told me to call her or a friend, or take a deep, soothing breath. Maybe nothing would have been different. I wondered if Cyree, Stella, Queenie, and Jonie believed their daughters would make different choices when they were confronted with the emotional impact that comes with sexual longing. I wondered what type of future circumstances might cause my son to ignore my warnings about responsibilities and safety. While I knew that I wouldn't have answers to these questions right away, I knew that in time we would all have the opportunity to see if our children had actually heard our messages. It seemed that we had all found a way to have God in our lives, but the struggle was still on in terms of our children. In the meantime listening and talking to my sister friends had helped me to remove a few more articles from my own emotional baggage.

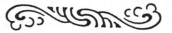

I AM NOT MY MOTHER'S DAUGHTER

The first fight I ever had with a man, I lost. The man was my older brother, and we were arguing about which television program we would watch. He wanted to see *The Twilight Zone* and I wanted to watch *The Flintstones*—both programs came on the same night, at the same time, and herein lay the problem: different channels. The political jockeying began at the dinner table.

"Momi, can I have my bath first? I want to be through by the time *The Flintstones* come on."

"Nobody wants to watch that dumb show; besides, tonight's Friday and *Twilight Zone* comes on."

"Both of you hush and eat. You know better than to argue at the table."

We hushed up only to eat hurriedly, giving each other looks designed to intimidate, and the countdown began. Later, freshly bathed and situated on the couch, I felt secure in my knowledge that at the appointed hour I would be permitted to turn to channel seven and watch my favorite show. Well, the hour arrived and I got up to turn the channel, only to be met with the low deep voice of my brother warning me not to touch that dial.

"We're watching *The Flintstones,* Momi said," I threw back over my shoulder as I continued to march toward the television set.

"She did not," my brother hissed, "and if you turn that channel I'll hurt you"—this last part just loud enough for my ears alone.

"Momi," I yelled, trying to rally some support in the face of danger, "didn't you say I could watch *The Flintstones?*" No response. "Momi," I yelled again, in the hope that she would come running to my aid as my brother advanced on me and pushed me away from the set.

"You all stop that noise before you wake up the other kids. If you're going to fight I'll turn that thing off and send both of you to bed. Now cut it out, Julia Anne." (Momi always used first and middle names when she meant business.) "If I hear your mouth one more time you're going to bed right now, do you hear me?" This was clearly not the response I was looking for, and since I wasn't ready to go to bed, I retreated back to the couch, but not before taking a swing at my brother, who grinned slyly as he settled in. I attributed my loss to several things. My brother was seven years older, physically bigger and stronger, and he had the privilege of being male in a (Southern) household that respected male authority. As a child I was constantly told by my mother to listen to and mind my older brother. Since I was born to question authority, I felt it was my inalienable right to ask why whenever I felt the sting of unfairness in a given situation. Without hesitation my question was always met with the parental reasoning of "He's older, that's why" or "He's your brother."

The implied message of his being male wasn't lost on me and in many ways the unspoken assumption helped to set the tone for my adult encounters with men when it came to conflict and confrontation. From that first lost argument with my brother over a television program, I learned that being male meant having a certain amount of authoritative power. I began to notice that my mother often made statements like "I'll have to talk it over with Daddy first" or "Let's see what Daddy has to say" or "Ask your father; if he says it's okay then it's okay with me too." I also noticed that many of the requests or decisions we asked Momi to make only got deferred to Daddy when he was home from one of his many business trips, leading me to believe that my mother had power too, but she was only willing to use it when Daddy wasn't present.

Momi was born in Augusta, Georgia, and raised in Baltimore, Maryland, in a household where both parents were wage earners, but the man always had authority in the home; this form of home training had a very strong influence on my mother's view of relationships, which she tried to pass on to her daughters. I learned from my mother that it was proper (Momi was a very traditional and proper Southern Black woman in many ways) and expected that a lady defer to her husband on matters of the home front. That's not to say that she and Daddy didn't disagree, because I wit-

nessed my share of knock-down-drag-out hassles between those two, but in the end Momi generally would
listen to my father's reasoning. And over the years,
Daddy became wise enough to know which issues not
to challenge my mother on.

I also learned something important about myself
during that first argument with my older brother. I
would stand up to authority and even take a swing at
it every now and then, but when the pressure was on
and my support was low I would retreat until I could
find a way to make myself heard.

Looking back on it, these early rounds with my older
brother provided an interesting backdrop for what occurred during my marriage. My husband had quite
conventional ideas about spousal relations and in the
beginning, trying to be the proper wife (and also being
young, and, I like to believe, naive), I accepted his
logic without question. After all, I reasoned, I wanted
to be like my mother, a good wife, and to do that I had
to keep peace and harmony in my marriage. My ex-
husband and I rarely argued, mainly because he acted
on whatever decision he made and generally told me
about it afterward, and as he so candidly told me in
the beginning of our relationship, I could either accept
it (his decision) and get mad, or not accept it and get
mad; either way it was up to him. But as I moved more
into a place of self-growth and discovery I started taking figurative swings at this form of subtle control by
following his example. I started making my own decisions, and then telling him about them. "Why didn't
you ask me first?" he would inquire. "You never ask
me about decisions that you make," I would respond,

and the argument was on. Sometimes I felt the need for support and called Momi, but as it was with my brother when I was younger, Momi would reply in a soft voice, "Well now baby, he is your husband." Again, not the response I wanted or needed to hear. Leaning on her own home training for guidance, my mother saw my husband as the voice of authority in our home. I knew deep down that as much as she loved me, Momi would never really understand or sanction the fact that I had started discovering my own voice. Sometimes when my husband and I could talk rationally about things he would state his concern about the changes I was making in myself. "You never acted like this before; you're changing and I don't know if I like it." In all fairness, he was right. I was changing, and while I wasn't sure if I totally embraced all the aspects of my changes, at that time in my life, I did know that I wanted to experience and enjoy a certain kind of emotional freedom.

"What type of emotional freedom are you talking about?" he would ask suspiciously.

"I'm not really sure, but I don't want to give up learning about and expressing myself. I'd really like to have your support, not your approval or disapproval, but just some support."

We were divorced a year later. Enough said.

In all honesty there were other things that played into that decision, but the main reason that stands out for me is that my movement in the struggling to be heard and acknowledged was the beginning of the breakdown of my marriage. Could I have changed it, taking back my voice? In the beginning I tried, but as some great prophet said, once one's eyes have been opened they can never be closed. I'm not going to lie— letting go of my marriage was one of the hardest experiences in my life, but I just wasn't willing to give up my voice.

> *I hate gettin' into fights with DeWayne 'cause I swear that man can hold a grudge better than anybody I know. He'll walk around for days not speaking and no matter what we fight about I always end up giving in 'cause I can't stand it when he won't talk to me.*
>
> *Jonie*

How did you settle the issue of not wanting to have another baby, Jonie? Because I remember you said that no matter what DeWayne said, you weren't going to give in on that one.

> *I'm not giving in on that one, and DeWayne knows it too. I just told him that we'll have to part company if he keeps pushing the issue. I love DeWayne and he knows that, but I made it clear the first time he brought it up that I just wasn't willing to give in on that subject, and my saying no doesn't mean I don't love him, it just means that I'm serious. I've given in to other stuff that he wanted just to keep the peace and to prove my commitment, but Arletta's almost a teenager and it's time for me to start paying some attention to some of the things I want. Every now and*

then he still brings it up, but I figure that's just his way of testing my willpower.

Jonie

I don't mind letting Willie run things 'cause most of the time he's right and I trust his judgment. But he knows he's got to let me have my say on something cause if he don't, I just fuss for days. I generally let him have his way as long as he lets me have my say.

Queenie

What if Willie wanted you to have another baby, Queenie, would you give in on that one?

Ella

Child, hush, Willie ain't no fool and unless he's planning to get pregnant and raise it by hisself he knows better than to even think that way. Besides, we're both too old to be thinkin' about raising anything except our old tired butts outta the bed.

Queenie

Marcus and I used to fight all the time when we first got together. If I said something was black he said it was white; we just couldn't seem to agree on nothing no matter how small it was. I could always tell when I was getting the better of him, 'cause he'd go off on this thing about how I didn't respect him as a Black man and the head of the family. Then he'd say that if he couldn't be the head of his house then he would just leave and I could make all the decisions, 'cause he wasn't gonna let no woman rule him. We actually broke up a couple of times before we finally got it together. Sometimes I would have to ask myself why in the world I was staying with him.

Stella

What helped you to hang in there with him, Stella?

Well, for one thing I knew Marcus loved me and I know I love him and the good times outmeasured the bad times. Plus neither one of us wanted to split up the family. At first I tried just keeping my mouth shut but I knew that wouldn't work 'cause I found myself building up resentments, and I would do stuff like withholding sex, 'cause I felt it was the only power play I had in my corner. But after our second breakup I took the baby, 'cause Renee was about three years old at the time, and I went to stay with Mama and told her everything, and she suggested that maybe we needed to talk to somebody to see if we couldn't come to some kind of understanding for the baby's sake. At first when I asked Marcus about seeing somebody he said no, 'cause he didn't want anybody in our business, especially some stranger. But then I told him I just couldn't come back and have things continue on the way they were going, so unless he could come up with something better, I was gonna take the baby and leave him for good. Well, honey, a few days later Marcus called and told me he would go talk to somebody with me. Well, to make a long story short, we went and talked to this therapist and she had us take this couple's class. We learned communication skills and something they call "fair-fighting skills." At first Mar-

cus didn't want to do it, and I admit I had my share of doubts too, but we stuck it out and we both were surprised because some of that stuff really works. Actually Marcus reminds me to use our skills when things start getting heated between us.

Stella

I'm really glad the two of you stuck it out, Stella, and got some help. I've discovered that a lot of arguments can be avoided when two people know how to communicate. Using skills like making "I" statements, as in, "I need to take a time out on this discussion"; listening and acknowledging your partner's statements with one- or two-word phrases like "I see" or "I'm listening"; giving feedback such as "I understand that you see the situation like this. Here's how I see the problem"; or making a plan to get back to the problem after taking some time to cool down, by stating, "I really can't talk about this now, I'm much too upset. Give me about twenty minutes to think this through and I'll get back to you with my response." Techniques like these can really make a big difference in how couples resolve disagreements. I often wonder what might have become of my marriage if we had known about and used some of these skills or had something like couple's communication classes.

Well, personally I hate the whole idea of fighting with someone you love. I used to watch my parents really go after each other. Calling each other names, throwing things, and hitting each other, all that mess really scared me when I was growing up, and then what I really didn't understand is, the next day they would be all lovey-dovey like nothing ever happened. I told myself that I wasn't ever going to fight with my partner 'cause it just wasn't worth it to me. Me and La-Shay have only been together for a couple years, but knock on wood we've agreed on most of the important stuff and when we don't agree we negotiate.

Nonie

I agree, Nonie, fighting is hard on any relationship, but realistically couples are going to disagree and argue from time to time. I think sometimes we have this expectation that just because we love someone, we're never going to disagree with that person, but when you have two people coming together from different backgrounds, with different values and beliefs, things get heated sometimes. Even when people share all those things—love, backgrounds, values, and beliefs—they're going to disagree at times. My brother and I were perfect examples of that one. Some disagreement can be healthy and even arguing can be beneficial when it's done constructively. I get concerned when arguments cross the line and turn into abuse or violence. Nothing gets resolved when couples engage in name-calling, personal attacks, and hitting. Those types of behavior are emotionally and physically dangerous to both parties.

When Phil and I first got together, we used to do what I call search and rescue. I would get mad about something and grab the boys, call a taxi 'cause I didn't know my way around the city when we first moved here, and go to a hotel and hole up there till Phil found us. Poor Phil, he would spend hours calling all over town looking for me and the kids. After the first couple of times, he caught on that I wouldn't go to my friends. He started calling hotels till he found us; by that time I had cooled down enough to talk, and he'd come to the hotel and rescue us and we'd end up spending the night together. Well, about a year ago, when we really got into it about something, he came to the hotel and told me that the next time we had an argument either I could stay and talk it out or get a hotel room on the East Coast, 'cause he wasn't going to keep calling all over town and coming to rescue me. I told him that I would be willing to talk it out if he would at least listen to me sometime. So far so good— the last time I spent the night in a hotel we checked in together.

Gracie

Well, you know what I hate, I just hate it when De-Wayne and I fight about something without solving the problem and then he expects to go to bed with me and make love like nothing ever happened. I don't know about the rest of you, but I can't fight one minute and make love two minutes later like nothing ever came down between us.

Jonie

You know, we talked about that in our communciation skills class, and what Marcus and I learned to do when we couldn't reach an agreement by bedtime, we agreed to table the discussion till the next day. And then the therapist told us to set a time during the day when we would come back to whatever we were arguing about and either reach some kind of understanding or agree to disagree. Now that was one that I didn't think would work, knowing Marcus the way I do, but the couple of times when we've done it, it's worked. We don't necessarily make love after we table the argument but at least we don't go to bed mad at each other.

Stella

Me and Winyah do that a lot, that agreeing to disagree on something. But Winyah has good skills in that area, because he works with those street kids and he uses communication skills with them.

Roxy

One of the most valuable things I learned after I'd divorced and started dating was the concept of agreeing to disagree at some point. I've also learned that after about the third date with someone, if it looks like we're going to be spending more time together, I ask him how he deals with his anger. Because if we continue to spend extended amounts of time together, we're bound to disagree on something, and I want to know what to expect. I also tell him how I deal with my anger so he'll know what to expect from me.

What if they don't know how they handle their anger? Better yet, what if you don't know how you handle your stuff?

Nonie

I believe that we all have a pretty good idea of how we handle our emotions; we may not always be clear about how we'll handle a new situation when it comes up. But by and large we've had enough experience with anger in our lives to know pretty much how we deal with it. I handle my anger in a couple of different ways. If I feel safe in a situation, my first response is to want to verbally defend why I'm taking a certain position. If I don't feel safe in a situation I'll do what I did as a child and retreat by withdrawing into myself for a period of time. Sometimes but not always I'll throw myself into a project as a way of mentally and emotionally working to forget the issue. If he tells me that he doesn't know how he handles his anger, or he's never really thought about it, I ask him to think about it and get back to me. If he says something like, "You'll find out when you make me angry" or "I don't get mad," I make tracks in the opposite direction because I consider those two responses red flags for potential danger.

What do you mean when you talk about being in a "safe situation" and "red flags" for danger?

Cyree

For me, Cyree, being in a safe situation means that I know enough about the person that I'm dealing with to trust his reactions in an emotional encounter or conflict. I have a couple of ways to gauge his emotional temperament. I listen to how a person talks about his day at the office or some other daily situation that he's been involved in. I'm listening to how the person describes and responds to his coworkers and how he has reacted to different types of stressful situations that may have come up. If I notice that he tends to frequently use negative, scornful, or derogatory words or remarks when describing or talking about others, that's my first clue as to how he views people. If he often sees stressful situations as being caused by someone else or if everything he encounters becomes a crisis, then that's my clue as to how he deals with situations. The other thing I do that proves to be really helpful is to watch how that person interacts with other people, whether he knows them or not. Is he friendly, polite, respectful, considerate? Does he appear to be comfortable engaging with others, without having to be the center of attention? Listening and watching may seem like small things, but both of these behaviors can provide you with a lot of useful information. When someone tells me he doesn't know how he handles his anger, that automatically puts me on guard as far as interacting with him, because like I said, if we plan on spending any time together there are going to be times when we disagree, and some people handle the challenge of disagreement in violent ways.

Yeah, my first husband was one of those. I still can't hear good in my right ear 'cause he got mad about something I said once, and he slapped me so hard it messed up my ear.

Gracie

What'd you say, Gracie?

Jonie

I told him to get the "f" outta my face, 'cause he was screaming at me about being late picking him up from work.

Gracie

Oooh, Gracie, I didn't know you knew words like that with your proper schoolmarm self.

Jonie

Shoot, girl, when the heat's on you'd be surprised at what words I know. I'm just glad me and Phil don't go through that kind of mess—once was enough for any sane person. Phil's more of a talker; honey, that man will talk you to death "just trying to understand," as he says. He knows that I have my moods and he tries to get me to talk about what's bugging me when I get in one of them. But now he knows that when I get like that the best thing to do is to let me be and I'll come around on my own. I can generally tell when something's bothering him 'cause he'll go running or spend time in his workshop hammer-and-sawing all night long. If it's something between us he's more likely to say let's talk, which generally means he needs to talk. And I'm going to do a lot of listening, but that doesn't mean that I have to agree with what he has to say.

Gracie

89

I'm glad you mentioned listening, Gracie, because as far as communication goes, listening is just as important as talking. I think that sometimes we get so caught up in wanting and needing to be heard that we forget the value of listening.

I don't mind listening, but if I don't say something, then DeWayne thinks I'm in agreement with him and sometimes I'm not.

Jonie

Do like I do, Jonie. Say something like "Yeah, baby, I hear you" every once in a while just to let them know that you're tuned in. Whenever I do that with Marcus, he'll end up sayin' something like "What do you think, baby?" And I'll tell him what I'm thinking.

Stella

Willie just lets me fuss; he'll say, "Go on and get it outta your system." 'Cause he knows I'm gonna fuss anyway, but then I'm gonna give in. But tell me something, sis. Do you ever wish that you hadn't given up on your marriage? I mean, couldn't you have just worked around him? I do that with Willie every now and then. But I figure it ain't worth it to lose my man over petty stuff.

Queenie

Do I miss my marriage? Yes, sometimes I do. But do I regret my decision? No, I don't regret it. As much as I loved my husband at the time, I was starting to love myself. It's a lot easier to say what could have been now that I know what my life is, but at that time I was scared to death. As I said, I wanted my marriage to work, but I also recognize that it takes two people to work at a relationship; he wasn't willing to give up who he was, and I wasn't willing to give up who I was becoming. I don't believe that people have to sacrifice their relationships because they can't communicate, but sometimes it happens.

When I think about the relationships I've been in and out of, I think about all the time I invest in trying to make it work. At some point it generally hits me that if the relationship was so good I wouldn't have to work so hard. It always seems like I'm the one making all the changes in my life and I start resenting the guy for not wanting to make the same kind of changes.

Ella

Preach on those resentments, Ella. 'Cause, honey, I got my list and I'm checkin' it twice.

Zoey

In my case, my changing was for the best. Gettin' back into the church, becomin' involved in the neighborhood, and not runnin' in the streets so I could raise my child right has really helped me be a better woman. Willie is older and he's been around the block a couple of times, that's why I trust him like I do, and I was willing to do whatever I needed to do in order to hold on to him, and that included changing my ways. He told me from the git-go that if I wanted to be with him then I had to get my life together, 'cause he wasn't interested in no woman that was more interested in runnin' the streets than she was in him.

Queenie

Don't get me wrong. I don't think making changes is wrong, but there has to be flexibility in order to allow the change to happen. The perfect solution would be if both parties made changes at the same time and were going in the same direction, but that's rare if it ever happens at all. Usually one person makes some changes in his or her life, and then there's a period of adjustment, and then maybe the other person starts making changes.

I was a little older than most of you all when I got married, so I was a little more settled in my ways. Winyah is younger than me, but when we met he had everything I was looking for in a man. He's a people person, he likes to talk, he's kind of like Gracie's Phil in that way, and he's gentle and kind. When he first asked me to marry him I struggled for a while with the age thing 'cause he's ten years younger, but then I thought, Shoot! Why not—he has everything I want, and if he's willing so am I. I kind of like it that he likes to talk things out between us, because it lets me know he's interested in what I'm thinking. And in the relationship department that was a first for me.

Roxy

Every now and again in one of my more reflective moments I think about my marriage and play the "what
if" game. What if I had just let him continue to make
all of the decisions, what if I had ignored my need to
grow and make changes in my life, what if he had
been more willing to be flexible, what if I had been
more willing to continue being the traditional type of
woman he wanted. When I add up all the what-ifs I
always come to the same outcome—No Way. When I
look at my life now, I realize that giving in a little
would have meant sacrificing a lot in terms of moving
forward with my life. Mama, my grandmother, once
told me, "Baby, you're gonna have to fight a lot in this
world; you're a Black woman, and our lives ain't never
been easy. Now some of us are gonna go to war about
every little thing, but I want you to remember to
choose your struggles real careful, make sure you're
fightin' for somethin' you really want 'cause you don't
want to wear yourself out over nothin'. But once you
make up your mind to fight for somethin' I want you
to give it every ounce of your breath, and fight like
there's no tomorrow 'cause you aim to win."

Well, in the case of my decision about my marriage,
I think Mama would have been proud. I chose my
struggle because I needed to be heard, I fought the best
fight I knew how, and as painful as the fight was, I
survived.

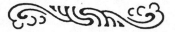

HAVING SOME FUN TALKING TRASH

Okay, everybody, the food's ready. Grab a plate and dig in.

Nonie, what kind of sauce is this on the chicken? It sure smells good.

Thanks, Zoey, it's a Thai sauce—try a little piece first 'cause it's kind of spicy.

Honey, there's two things in this world that can't be spicy enough, my chicken and my men.

Oh, Lord, here she goes.

I was just telling the truth, Ella honey, it ain't nothing but the truth.

Well, since you're into telling the truth, Miz Zoey, can I ask you a personal question?

Go for it, sweetcakes. Ella, if I had known you'd be bringing greens I would've whipped up a batch of corn bread.

Okay, when was the last time you had absolutely incredibly good sex?

Hold up, sis. Let me put my chicken down, 'cause I don't want nothing in my mouth when I hear this one. Go 'head, Zoey, spit it out girl.

Sis, why you want to mess with me when I'm eatin'? Is this gonna end up on the front page of some international tabloid exposé that you buy at the supermarket checkout stand?

Come on, Zoey, you said you'd answer sis—what's the juice girl?

Look at you, Stella, just dipping all in my Kool-Aid.

Let's hear it, Zoey, don't go acting all shy. What's the scoop?

Now, Roxy, you ain't never known me to be shy about nothin'. But you know the old saying, When you kiss and tell you dry up the well. But if you must know it was this morning and I'm here to tell you it was so good till it made my toes curl. There! Now are you satisfied? Pass the hot sauce, sis.

What made it so good for you, Zoey?

That depends. Do you want facts or details? Queenie, pass me them rolls.

Zoey, girl, you're somethin' else. Sis, you wanna put some more rolls in the oven? I just gave Zoey the last one.

Come on, Zoey. Fess up—what made this time better than before?

Sis, you might as well skip on over me with your questions, 'cause I ain't sayin' another word till I finish this plate. Stella, girl, you put your whole foot in these black beans, honey, you have outdone yourself.

Gracie, baby, can you get me the salad dressing while

you're up. Zoey may not be talkin' but, honey, I don't know what got into Mr. Leon last night, 'cause when I got home from work he had fed the kids, got them ready for bed, and fixed me dinner. And are you ready for this—while I was eatin', brother man even ran me a hot bath, bubbles and all. Now if you don't think I didn't invite him to join me in the tub . . .

Cyree, girl, you need to hush.

Come on, Queenie, you and Willie been together forever. You mean to tell me you all don't be knockin' the boots?

Now, I didn't say all that; it's just that in the beginning when we were new to each other Willie took a little more time than he does now. I mean, well let's just put it this way, what he used to do all night, well now it takes him all night to do. But what he does do is just fine, thank you very much.

Ahh! suckey, suckey now, go 'head on with your bad self, Miz Queenie.

You hush, Jonie. Hangin' out with you all done made me forget myself for a minute there. Sis, you better check on those rolls. I smell somethin' burnin'.

Winyah's been wantin' me to check out one of those strip joints with him. I have to admit I'm kind of curious, but I'd probably be the only woman sittin' up in there with all my clothes on.

You should check it out. Roxy, me and DeWayne went to one and it wasn't half bad. Honey, I even learned a few new moves. Here, let me show you one. Hey, sis, you got any spare tassels layin' around?

Jonie, sit your wild butt down, girl. Is there any more rice?

I've never been to one of the men's clubs before, but me

and a bunch of girls from my office checked out that new club Big Daddies over in midtown. Child, I surprised myself, I was screaming and yelling so loud till I was hoarse for two days. Those dudes were some kind of fine; I break out in a cold sweat just thinkin' 'bout them. Nonie, hand me that glass, I'll take it to the kitchen.

Stella, girl, were they fine?

Child, I ain't gonna lie, those dudes were so fine till they brought tears to my eyes. I've already decided I'm givin' Marcus a membership to the gym for his birthday, and for Christmas I'm buyin' him a couple pair of bikini briefs and guess who he's gonna unwrap for New Year and I don't plan to be wearin' no diaper and sash neither.

Stella, girl, you're too crazy.

I don't know about those places, seems to me like all they do is make women look like trash. Men exploit women enough without us helping them.

Oh, come on, Nonie, they ain't all that bad. I would rather see women in a place like that gettin' paid than out on the street workin' for some lowlife pimp.

Well, what's the difference? If you ask me it's all the same thing, they're either shakin' their asses on a table or they're shakin' them on the street.

Zoey, pass that hot sauce on over here.

I don't think it's the same thing at all, Queenie; at least the sister in the club gets to keep the money she makes. Shoot, if push came to shove and I had to feed myself and Arletta, and didn't have any other means of makin' it, I could see myself dancin' in a club.

Jonie! What are you saying? It's exploitation either way. Don't you know what goes on in those places—drugs, racketeering, you name it.

Watch your blood pressure, Nonie, Jonie is just talkin'. Actually I don't see why you all are gettin' so upset. Frankly speakin', I think that on both counts the sisters are makin' choices. In my opinion neither choice is all that good, but when it comes right down to it the bottom line is always gonna be survival.

You make it sound so easy, Zoey. But I agree with Nonie, we've just got to start makin' better choices for ourselves as women.

I agree with you, Cyree; we do have to look at makin' better choices for ourselves. All I'm sayin' is that the truth of the matter for some of us, and I know it's a shame to say it, workin' in the sex trade is sometimes the lesser of a lot of the evils that we have goin' on in our lives. Who left this teaspoonful of rice in the bottom of the bowl? Sis, where's your rice and a saucepan? I'll make us up some more.

Well, you'll never guess where I went the other day. Stella, I want the recipe for this pasta salad.

Get your head out the bowl, Ella, and tell us where you went, girl.

I went to the Rubber Tree, you know, that new sex shop over on Broadway.

No you didn't, Ella, I don't believe it, with your proper-never-miss-church-on-Sunday self. Child, you gonna have a whole heap of testifyin' to do come Sunday mornin'.

Don't even go there, Queenie, 'cause I may be in the church but I ain't no saint yet. Anyway, I knew I was gonna be kickin' it with my friends on Saturday night and I didn't want to be caught off guard, you know what I mean.

Git on down, Miz Ella, with your bad self.

Dottie, this girl at my office just kept talkin' 'bout the

Rubber Tree having all kinds of good stuff and all, so I just thought I'd sneak a peek. Well, honey! I'm here to tell you they got everything in that store from A to Z. I'm talkin' movies, books, chains, feathers, whips—you name it, they got it. I saw my first dildo and I'm thirty-five years old. I was so busy lookin' till I almost forgot what I went in there for.

What did you go in there for? I just want to know so I get all the facts right. I don't wanna leave nothin' out when I pray for your sorry behind soul on Sunday.

Hush, Queenie. Girl, what'd you buy?

Some condoms and K-Y jelly. What'd you think I was gonna buy? I started to get a pair of handcuffs, you know, just for fun, but I thought it'd be just my luck for some fool to rob me and leave me handcuffed to a tree somewhere.

Did you see any ben-wa balls? I read this story where this girl used ben-wa balls and I was wondering what they were.

Gracie, I saw some of everything and I probably saw those too. But to be real honest I didn't know half of what I was lookin' at, and I didn't think it would be a good idea to ask, know what I mean.

When LaShay and I first started going out we used to go to the Rubber Tree all the time. I like all the different kinds of lotions and body rubs.

Nonie, you a little young to be having sex aren't you? Okay, okay, girlfriend, don't roll your eyes at me. I was just kiddin'. Stella, could you pour me another glass of wine while you're up? Thanks.

I know I look young but remember I'll be twenty-four in two months. Shoot, me and Shay been together almost two years. Hey, Ella, do your condoms glow in the dark?

Nonie! What kind of freakish mess is that?

It's true, Queenie, they have all kinds of condoms in that place. And no, baby girl, I just bought the plain old everyday kind.

Ebonie, you're being awful quiet over there. I know you're just visitin', sis, but don't be shy, girlfriend; we talk crazy trash like this all the time. So feel free to jump in at any time. Do you want some more chicken?

Thanks, Cyree, I feel real comfortable with you all. It's just that I might not have too much to add to this conversation because, well, let's just say I'm practicing celibacy right now.

Girl, what's to practice? Or is that the new polite way of sayin' you ain't got a man in your life at the moment? Can somebody bring that bowl of fruit and platter of cheese over here from the table.

Jonie! Child, leave Ebonie alone, just 'cause you all put your business in the street. You have to excuse them, baby; they get a little carried away every now and then.

No, it's okay, Queenie, I'm really enjoying myself. To answer your question, Jonie, well, let's just say I'm not having partnered sex at the moment. But my fantasies do manage to keep me busy and very satisfied.

Honey, I just can't get with that self-pleasuring as they so politely call it nowadays.

Actually, Roxy, some people find masturbation or self-pleasuring to their sexual fantasies quite satisfying. In fact a lot of folks are calling it the "new sex." Masturbation, celibacy, and flirting openly for pleasure have been around for centuries. We can call them new but I think folks are just rediscovering other ways of being sexual.

Well, that ain't what I'd call them.

What would you call them, Queenie?

I can tell you in short order. The first one is nasty, the second one is a shame, and third is playin' games. Pass the pound cake.

Queenie, I swear, girl, you've got to come out of the dark ages. Don't you ever have sexual fantasies?

Yeah, I used to have them till I found out that Michael Jordan didn't make house calls. Anyway, what do I need to fantasize about—I got Willie, and like I told you, he takes care of business just fine. Besides, I'm from the old school. Sex should be private—you start puttin' your business in the street and the next thing you know somebody will come along and pick it up.

Well, honey, I'm from the new school and I want to know everything—maybe if I put enough business out there I'll get some.

Ella, child, I swear you are some kind of wild. Your prince is coming, just give him some time.

Yeah, well, he better hurry up or I'm going to end up dying from DTS.

Girl, what in the world . . . ?

It stands for dry twat syndrome.

You know, Ella, there are other options available to you. Good sex doesn't always have to involve two people.

Lord have mercy Jesus! Let me put this plate down and get my coat, 'cause if she starts talkin' 'bout havin' sex with animals I'm out the door.

I hear you, Queenie. I'll be right behind you, 'cause I may be horny but I damn sure ain't crazy.

Well, I wasn't going to, but since you mention it. No! Wait, you two, I was only kidding. Actually I was thinking about what Ebonie had mentioned earlier, you know, self-pleasuring. There are a lot of great sex toys out there designed to help a woman enhance her own sexual pleasure.

Thank you, Father, 'cause I was just about ready to go to church and light up every candle in the place for you, sis.

Am I that bad, Queenie?

I'll put it to you like this, girlfriend. You've been known to wander off from the mother ship every once in a while to orbit places unknown.

Queenie, you're too much. Sis is right, Ella; they have quite a few things for women in that sex store that you went to for your condoms. I know because I've gotten a few goodies for myself there.

Stop, Zoey, you've been to the Rubber Tree. But you've always got some man swinging from your arm.

Well, let's just put it this way, sometimes I'm my own best company in the sex-for-pleasure department.

I've always wondered if people really used that stuff.

Somebody must use it, or they wouldn't have a store selling it.

My friend Blanche invited me to a women's-only erotic party one time, and I won a pair of edible panties. Well, honey, I couldn't wait to get home and try them out on Leon. So I go home, hop in a nice hot shower, dry myself off, and put these panties on in that hot steamy bathroom. Well, child, before I could get from the bathroom to the bedroom I started feelin' this sticky goo runnin' down my legs—child, the panties started meltin'. Leon and I were laughing so hard till we were cryin'. Here I thought I was goin' to be a sex kitten and I turned out bein' a sticky, gooey lollipop for my baby.

Cyree, you mean Leon licked it off?

You think he didn't, baby? We really had a good time that night.

Girl, that reminds me of the time I was trying to be cute and make like Lady Godiva with this real long wig. I lit all these candles around the bed and put on this really soft music. Child, I was gonna give DeWayne the night of his life. I'm sittin' straddlin' his back just a rubbin' with all this long hair hangin' down, I mean I'm really into it. After a few minutes DeWayne said, "Baby, I smell something burning." And me tryin' to be all sexy and keep the mood told him, "Oh baby, that's just my burnin' passion you smell." DeWayne said, "No baby, really, I smell something burning for real," and just when he said that, I noticed this black smoke puffin' up from the side of the bed and DeWayne started screamin', "Baby, your hair's on fire! Your hair's on fire!" Girl, I snatched that wig off so fast I got dizzy. You should have seen us, I'm standin' up there naked to the world stampin' out my wig, and DeWayne's running around the room buck naked blowin' out candles. Between the smoke from the wig and all those candles being blown out, the smoke alarm went off and shook us up so bad till we couldn't find the button to turn it off. Somebody downstairs must have called the fire department 'cause the next thing we knew we heard all these sirens. All

I can say is we must have looked like two crazy fools standin' up there in our bathrobes tryin' to explain to all those firemen and the department manager how it was just a mistake. To this day I can't pass a firehouse without blushing.

Jonie, stop please, don't say another word. I can't stand it. Ebonie baby, hand me that napkin over there.

Girl, I swear it's true. Poor DeWayne cringes every time he sees a woman with long hair.

Well, honey, Mr. Marcus really surprised me about a month ago. Apparently he'd seen me reading this article in Essence *magazine on sexual fantasies and he asked me if I ever fantasized about making love to anybody other than him. At first I said no and just left it alone. But he kept bugging me, so I told him that every once in a while I did fantasize about bein' in a club and havin' a tall dark stranger approach and sweep me off my feet. Well, you all know Marcus, he's kind of quiet and you never really know what he's thinkin', so when he didn't say any more about it I figured he just forgot about it. Well, 'bout a couple weeks later I get this call from him at work and he asked me to meet him downtown at Maxi's for dinner. So I got all dressed up and went thinkin' we'll have dinner and I'll talk him into taking me to a late movie. When I got to Maxi's, Marcus wasn't nowhere to be found so I had the waiter show me to a table thinkin' that maybe Marcus had got caught in traffic and was runnin' late. I sat at that table for a good fifteen minutes by myself, callin' Marcus everything but a child of God under my breath, and just as I was gettin' ready to go find a phone to call his sorry butt, the waiter brought over this glass of wine and told me it was with compliments from the gentleman at the bar. I* looked over and there was Marcus big as life. Honey, he was decked out from head to foot; I swear he looked like he just stepped off the cover of GQ, and when he saluted me with his glass of wine you could have knocked me over with a feather. It was so romantic, like something in a movie. After about a couple of minutes of staring at me, he came over, introduced himself, and started flirting with me. I mean I just couldn't get over it. We had dinner, danced, and check it out, my baby had even reserved the bridal suite for us to spend the night. All I can say is I haven't felt so special in years.

Oh, Stella, that sounds so romantic, girl. Does Marcus have any brothers? Even a distant cousin will do.

Come on now, Ella, get a grip, girlfriend. Remember there's still the Rubber Tree.

I don't know, Zoey.

You know Zoey's right. I haven't said too much before but I feel kind of comfortable with you all so I'll just tell you all that I'm bisexual. I'm visiting sis right now because I just broke up with a woman I've been with for two years, and I needed a little vacation.

Gosh, Ebonie, I'm sorry to hear about your breakup, but I think I can speak for all of us when I say we're all pretty open-minded here when it comes to a person's sexual orientation. Even old crazy Queenie over there, ain't that right, Queenie?

You got that right, Jonie. They call me crazy, but most of the time I'm the sanest person around. I'm gonna get us all to heaven in one piece—that is, if I don't wear myself out prayin' for all their tired crazy butts. But I love 'em all.

You're in good company, sis. I'm a lesbian and I've been with my partner LaShay for almost two years now. She's *not here today because she's studying for a midterm. I'm really sorry to hear about your breakup. I think we've all been on that side of the street at some point in time.*

Ella, I just want to say that self-pleasuring can really be fun and enjoyable, if you get your imagination going.

I don't know, Ebonie, I guess I'm like Queenie in that department. I know what I like and what I want but when it comes to puttin' the two together I just go blank. Maybe something's wrong with me.

Let me assure you right now, Ella, there's nothing wrong with you. A lot of us share the inability to imagine ourselves in sensual, sexual situations. I recently read an article that stated that African American women had the least imagination when it came to sexual fantasies. Needless to say I think that magazine article was all wrong. I just think that we're the first generation of Black women to have the time or availability to really engage in this sort of pleasure so it's still new to us, and we may need a little help to get us started. First off I would suggest getting yourself some good erotic reading material. There are a number of good erotic books on the market, written by women for women on sexual erotica.

I can lend you a couple of my books, Ella.
Thanks, Zoey.

There are also a few women's erotic videos on the market. But I want to warn you right now, don't expect much of a plot or story line—these movies are centered on raw sex.

Sis, I'd like to add something if I may. I'm pretty uncomfortable with the movies I've seen, but that just has to do with my personal taste. But Ella, if you have a personal computer you might want to use your code name to hook into one of the Internet sex chat lines. They're kind of fun and I've found that doing that really helps to stimulate my senses.

That's a great idea, Ebonie. There are a number of things you can do to get your sensual senses stimulated. The other important thing that you may need to do is become comfortable with touching your body. I like the idea of using scented oils and lotions, massaging them slowly into your body starting at the scalp and working your way down to your neck, shoulders, breast, stomach, hips, genitals, and legs. Just go slow and feel your body relax as you massage each part of yourself.

Don't forget about the scented candles and soft music. Luther Vandross does it for me. Queenie, close your mouth, girlfriend, and watch that cup—you're about to spill punch all over the floor.

I don't know, it all sounds good but I don't know. Zoey, will you come with me if I decide to go back to the Rubber Tree?

Sure I will, sweetcakes. I need to replenish a few of my supplies anyway. I'll even take you over to Baby Dolls—that's a shop just for women.

I want to go too, Zoey.

So do I, girl. When are you all going?

You know this stuff sounds all well and good, but I had a pretty traumatic sexual experience when I was younger, and I don't want to go into details now; I've been getting some help and I'm starting to feel better about myself, but

I still have some hang-ups in the sex department. I mean Winyah, bless his heart, has been wonderful, he's done everything but stand on his head in the rain, and I think he'd do that too if he thought it would help, but for the life of me I can't orgasm. Winyah says it doesn't matter to him as long as I'm getting some kind of pleasure out of our lovemaking, and I do, but I don't want to feel like I'm cheating him out of anything.

I'm really glad that you and Winyah have such a caring, sensitive, and intimate relationship, Roxy. I think it shows a lot of respect and trust for you to be able to talk to him about your concerns, and it shows the same that he can care and understand what you're dealing with here. I'm not a real expert when it comes to talking about orgasmic responses, but I've read a number of articles by experts that state that an orgasm is not a measure of a woman's sexuality. In fact, from what I've read it seems that a woman's orgasmic response is still somewhat of a mystery to women and men alike. A number of experts acknowledge that they can provide straightforward clinical information regarding a woman's anatomy; however, it really comes down to a woman needing some form of sexual stimulation in order to achieve orgasm. Some women need manual or oral clitoral stimulation along with intercourse to achieve orgasm and others are so comfortable and know their bodies so well until they can orgasm just by having erotic thoughts. Several articles mentioned that women and some men may have a difficult time ever reaching orgasm due to childhood sexual trauma. However, all of the experts stated that orgasms aren't necessary in order to enjoy sex. It sounds to me like Winyah is interested in whether or not you're comfortable and able to enjoy some aspects of your lovemaking, which I might add is very sensitive of him. However, if you're bothered by not being able to achieve orgasm, then it might be a good idea to talk to a certified sex therapist to get more information.

You know, sis, once when LaShay was away on a business trip, I dreamed about her and woke up all wet.

In some circles, Nonie, that's what's known as a wet dream.

Get outta here, Zoey. Women can't have wet dreams, can they, sis?

Sure Nonie, Zoey's right—women can experience wet dreams too.

This may sound weird but when I was pregnant with Arletta I wanted it all the time. I used to follow Artis, that's Arletta's daddy, around like a puppy beggin' for scraps. He couldn't believe that I'd want to make love bein' pregnant. But for some reason it sure felt good to me then.

I was the same way, Jonie, when I was pregnant with Tyrone. But honey, when I got pregnant with Clayton I was sick as a dog, and the only thing I wanted then was to be left alone.

Some experts say that during pregnancy, we feel more emotional freedom, and can in fact enjoy lovemaking more than we do when we're concerned about whether or not we may get pregnant.

Well when we make our trip down to the sex shop, I'm gonna see if I can find something that will make DeWayne go down on me. I swear I've done everything but sit on his face to get him down there and he still refuses to budge.

Excuse me, but I'm trying to eat over here.

Oops, sorry, Queenie.

Jonie, if you give me a dollar I'll tell you how to get De-Wayne down there.

Zoey, you need to be shot—didn't we just finish talking about sexual exploitation? And for God's sake here's a napkin. Stop licking your fingers, it looks so dang nasty.

Ya! You're right, Stella. I forgot about that, okay. Jonie, keep the dollar, I'll tell you anyway. Girl, I don't know what you're talkin' about, I ain't wastin' none of this curry on a piece of paper, you'll just have to excuse my lack of home trainin' for a minute.

Stop messin' with her, Stella. So, Zoey, what's the secret?

Well, girlfriend, here's what you do. You get you some nice meaty chicken drumsticks, season 'em and fry 'em up real good and crispy and then hide them under your pillow. Then you take a nice hot bubble bath and towel yourself off and climb between the sheets. Take one of the drumsticks and rub a little of the grease behind your ears, and on your breast—you know the drill. Then stick it gently between your legs and call DeWayne. I guarantee you, boyfriend will eat from head to toe, suck the meat off the bone, and lick you dry lookin' for some more.

Girrrl! I don't believe you just said that. I swear, Zoey, you're somethin' else.

Queenie, you okay? You're looking a little green around the gills, girlfriend.

I'm okay, Ella. See you all sittin' over there laughin', just encouragin' Zoey to talk all this kind of mess. I swear she ain't nothin' but the devil.

I was just trying to help Jonie out is all. Girlfriend had a problem so I gave her a solution. Besides, it helps to be a little outrageous every once in a while.

Men don't seem to have a problem wantin' us to go down on them, but when it comes to them givin' us a little taste, child, they want to act like we're outta our minds.

Personally, Ella, I don't know if I want a man down there, and I'm not real sure I would like it. What if he don't know what he's doin'? No, thanks, I'll stick to what I know best—heads up.

Stella, honey, believe me, if they get that far, they'll know what they're doing. I remember the first time I asked Phil to go down on me, honey, you would have thought I asked him to swing naked from the Empire State Building. I mean brother man got real tight, but I explained to him—you know how Phil likes to understand everything—anyway, I just explained to him how good it made me feel, and then I gave him a little demonstration just so he'd get the idea. Then I told him, "Now you see, Phil, just like you screamed for mercy, I want to scream for a little mercy too." Brother man's been an active participant ever since.

Gracie, honey, you're too much.

I think I might have a little more luck with DeWayne using your approach, Gracie. With my luck I would end up frying and smelling like chicken only to have him give up eatin' meat. But thanks for the tip, Zoey.

Any time, sweetcakes.

Well, when we go to that store I want to make sure that I get something on fantasies. Ever since Marcus and I had that little adventure with my fantasy we've been sharing and playing out each other's fantasies. I'm gonna see if I can find a book on fantasies so we can get some more ideas.

Well, I want to see about gettin' some of those lotions and oils Nonie's been talking about.

How about you Queenie, do you want to come with us? We should all go together, it'll be fun.

No thank you, girlfriend, I'll just kind of do what I've been doin' all along. Willie ain't had no complaints and I don't have any so I'll stick with my original game plan.

I just want to check in with you Roxy. We got kinda deep there for a minute or two—how you doing, girl-friend?

I'm okay, sis; in fact, listening to you all has given me some ideas. When are you all going to that store?

How about you, Ebonie? Are you okay? We got kind of wild tonight.

Sis, I haven't had this much fun in a long time. Yeah, I'm fine—I'm kind of sorry I have to leave before you all go on your little field trip.

Don't worry, honey, the next time you come to town, we'll take you to all the hot spots. Maybe Nonie can fix you up with a blind date.

Ella, you're so bad. But if you're interested, Ebonie, I do know some nice single people.

Well, I'm not really ready for that yet, but who knows about later. I would love to come for another visit though.

Ebonie, you're welcome anytime girlfriend, any-time.

Sis, I'm in the mood for some tea. Where's your tea-kettle?

Nonie, can I take some of this chicken home? Come on over here and tell me how you make this sauce.

Gracie, girl, you'll never guess who I saw. . . .

Mama, my grandmother, used to say if you want to know what's on a person's mind or in his heart just set the table, 'cause folks don't lie on a full stomach. Every time I think I know it all, my sister friends show me in different ways just how much I have to learn about the whole concept of enjoying sex. My plate was filled several times over tonight as I listened to my sisters deal with the issue of sex with humor, sensitivity, and awareness. Sometimes we get so wrapped up in the day-to-day happenings we forget to laugh. I have a quote of Zora Neale Hurston's that I keep on my desk as a reminder that nothing in life is more important than my need to love and laugh at myself:

I Love Myself When I'm Laughing.

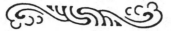

DATING AND MATING

There are two things that I dislike more than anything else on Mother Earth: snakes and being caught off guard. I don't camp, hike, or hang out in zoos, and I canceled my subscription to *National Geographic* ages ago, thereby lowering my chances of coming in contact with snakes. Now being caught off guard, that's another story altogether, and after my divorce (which was the ultimate being-caught-off-guard experience because I believed I would be married for life), I recognized the need to step up my vigilance in this area. Being bound and determined never to be caught in this type of situation again, I became a master list maker. As illogical as it sounds today, at that time I truly believed that scheduling every waking moment of every single day for the rest of my life would somehow keep me safe from the scary clutches of the unknown. I didn't want to think. Thinking was dangerous—I just wanted to do something, anything that would keep my mind off pain. Mastering the art of making and following a daily list of tasks during that period seemed to be the perfect solution.

I planned everything. A vacant moment in time meant a thoughtful moment, and my thoughts on being a single parent—emotionally vulnerable, financially unstable, and rejected by someone I had intended to love for the rest of my life—resembled the snakes that terrified me physically. I was afraid that if given time, my thoughts on my then-current state of affairs would poison and crush whatever spirit I had managed to cling to during the divorce. Raising my son, working two jobs to make ends meet, and attending graduate school kept my list pretty full for two solid years. And my list-making and -following abilities paid off big-time. I graduated and acquired one well-paying job in place of two lower-paying positions; and while my son (by now a budding teenager) still required my care and attention, it was to less of a degree.

My list for survival grew smaller and less demanding, leaving me with time to think about my life. Most of my thoughts about how to manage seemed less scary now, mainly because I had found a way to conquer them. All but one that is; the thought of being alone. When I stopped making lists I had time to look around, and I noticed that I was alone in a world that seemed populated by couples. I wasn't lonely in the traditional sense—I had an abundance of women friends who provided me with sisterly support and comfort, and like me, a few were single. The majority were married or in long-term relationships, though, and while they spoke of envying my so-called freedom, I noticed they guarded their relationships with a vengeance. I had only been single for two years, after a ten-year marriage, and didn't know what to expect. Everything I read or saw on television talk shows about the subject of being a single woman either scared me silly ("Single women are more likely to be victimized") or left me feeling hopeless ("Single women over the age of thirty are more likely to be hit by lightning than they are to marry").

This last report on the state of affairs for single women sent me running to the phone to call my friend Zoey. I'd known Zoey for years, and if anybody knew the real scoop on singles life it had to be her. And while I've never known her to be married (although she told me she was once "for a hot minute," as she put it), I've also never known her to be without companionship when she wants it. I've seen Zoey shop for a date, in much the same way I shop for shoes. Since we both tend to be pretty choosy about the quality of what we get, it would never occur to either one of us not to be prepared. I go shopping armed to the teeth with the triple C's—checkbook, credit cards, and cash—and Zoey's only form of ammunition is her firm determination that by the end of the evening she'll have a gentleman of her liking on her arm, ready, willing, and able to do her bidding. I knew that if anybody had a grip on the status of being a single woman in search of companionship it had to be Zoey.

"Zoey, I just heard some disturbing news about being single."

"You've been watching those talk shows again, haven't you?"

"Yeah! Well, you know how it is when you're folding clothes. Anyway, did you know that a single woman over thirty is more likely to get hit by lightning than she is to marry?"

"And the point of this enlightening survey, and your interest in it, is what?"

"Zoey, I don't want to spend the rest of my life alone. I want a relationship, maybe even to get married again. Don't you miss having someone special in your life, someone to love?"

"Everyone in my life is special, and you know me, I date when the mood strikes me. But as for the *L* word, well, I'm more inclined to believe in LWP."

"What in the world is LWP Zoey?"

"It stands for Lust With Potential, sis. At some point I might meet Mr. Right, but I don't intend to hold my breath until that point comes, know what I mean?"

"But don't you miss the sexual intimacy that comes with knowing a person for a while? And besides, casual sex can be dangerous not just physically, but emotionally. I don't know if I can handle LWP, Zoey. I wouldn't mind dating, but I would want it to lead to something more than a one-night stand."

"I hear where you're coming from sweetcakes—my particular style doesn't fit everyone. But I learned a long time ago that I was a lot happier being the one doing the choosing when it comes to my intimate needs than being the one chosen. Sure, I think about settling down with one person every once in a while, but it hasn't happened yet and I just don't want to take the time to worry about it. As for practicing safe sex, well, honey, you're preaching to the preacher on that one. Now do us both a favor and stop watching those damn TV talk shows."

Today when I think about my conversation with Zoey, I have to laugh. She thought I was gullible, which I was, when it came to believing the hype concerning being a single woman, and I thought she was naive, which she wasn't, when it came to making your own rules about relationships. What can I say? I've definitely learned a lot from that woman, the main lesson being to have a healthy dose of skepticism when it comes to surveys of any kind. I've also learned a great deal about myself from trial and error in the area of intimate relationships.

My first lesson on the dating and mating front came in the form of a tall, handsome, professional workaholic. We met on the phone during a business transaction, and I was immediately attracted to his no-nonsense approach to getting things done and his dry wit. After several telephone contacts we decided to meet in person and get to know each other.

To make a long story short, we found ourselves attracted to each other, and our six-year on-again, off-again relationship began. I fell in love and he just fell period. I fell in love because that's what I was used to, and that's what I wanted to do. This man had all the qualities I wanted in a person. He was intelligent, had a sense of humor, and loved his work, which took up a great deal of his time; and we were great in bed together.

My agenda was clear, even if it was only in my head: I wanted a lifetime committed partnership. Our communication was never explicit on this subject; however, I do remember hearing him say in the beginning of the relationship that he had problems with commitment because of his work demands. I heard but obviously I wasn't really listening, because I thought I could change him. To be honest, I don't know if he had an agenda and I never stopped to ask this important question, because I truly believed that once he knew how I felt about him he wouldn't be able to resist committing to a life together. I think that our relationship lasted six years and not longer because we were working from separate unspoken agendas. I told him how I felt but not what I wanted; he never said either way but operated on the assumption that what we had was enough and as good as it would get.

Riddle: how many times can a heart be broken? Answer: often, if it's not handled with care. I also learned something very important about myself in this relationship; I found that I was giving up bits and pieces of myself, parts that I had learned to start loving: making time to spend with friends and setting aside personal time for myself. I also refrained from talking about certain subjects—commitment or living together, for example—in order to avoid conflict. I never said no to him even when a request seemed unreasonable. He never directly asked me to give up these things, but I wanted this relationship to work, and I felt an unspoken pressure that to be the woman I thought he wanted me to be, I had to surrender certain parts of myself.

I'm not sure if the pressure was coming from him or me, but I would suspect that we both contributed in our own way: I contributed by not speaking up; he contributed by assuming everything was okay. The upside to this relationship was that we had dynamite sex, we never fought (mainly because we only saw each other for limited amounts of time and I didn't confront him on things), and we were sexually good together. Oh, I mentioned that earlier, but that was the best part of our relationship. Come to think about it, sex was our relationship, but like everything we chose not to talk about openly, this too was never really acknowledged. Now when I think about this relationship I recognize that while we both gained in the department of sexual gratification, that seems to be the only thing we gained equally in the time we spent together.

Excuse me, sis, but I've been sitting here wondering what in the world made you hang in there for so long. Good sex might be somethin' to write home about, but mercy, child, was it six years' worth of good?

Queenie

You know, Queenie, for a while I asked myself that same question, but finally I came to the conclusion that this relationship more than anything else was comfortable and it was easy. It was comfortable because I always knew what to expect and when to expect it, and the predictability of having sex on a regular basis made it easy. One of the things that I missed most about my marriage was having sex, and sharing that special closeness with another person.

My upbringing taught me that sex without love was wrong. I wanted guilt-free sex and I thought the only way to achieve it was by being in love. My lesson was in learning that one didn't have to be in love in order to enjoy sexual intimacy with another person. Now if you want to break it down in terms of numbers I figure it took me one year to learn that lesson and five years to get used to the idea.

I don't know what I'd do if Marcus ever said he wasn't in love with me anymore and wanted a divorce. He's the only man I've ever been with sexually and I think we're pretty good together in that way.

Stella

Honey, my hat is off to all my single sisters, 'cause I don't know if I could do it. If Winyah left me today or tomorrow I'd just go sign myself into the nearest convent. Ain't no need in me lying, as much as I like sex I ain't about to go through all the changes I watch all you single sisters go through.

Roxy

Well, I'm kinda like sis. I've learned a little more about myself every time I'm with somebody new. It's like I know I'm much less willing to put up with the same type of mess I put up with from men now than I was willing to deal with in my twenties. I mean, the brother's got to come to the table with something on his plate besides meat, 'cause I'm not willing to be nobody's side dish.

Ella

Dating and Mating

I've always wanted to be married and it took me two tries to get it right. Not just because of the sex but because I think I'm a better woman when I'm in a relationship. Maybe that sounds old-fashioned or somethin' but it's true for me. Me and my second husband, Carl, did good for a while, but things broke down somewhere along the line and I guess we just grew apart. But Phil, now that's another story—we both knew what we wanted when we came together and we just clicked. And to be real honest, sex with Phil isn't as exciting as it was with Carl, but there are other payoffs that I like better. I know I can always count on Phil to be there with and for me and the kids. Plus Phil and I share the same values about work, church, and family coming first, and we talk a lot to each other about different things, and I love that part of our relationship.

Gracie

I've learned a lot about myself in the years since my divorce; mainly I've learned that relationships are major responsibilities that require work on the part of both individuals.

When you say work, what do you mean, sis? 'Cause if you're talkin' about working around the house, me and Willie should've parted ways a long time ago. We ain't married but I've been with him for ten years, and, honey, the only thing that man picks up on a regular basis is the remote control. But I can say this much for him, he ain't missed a day's work at the post office since I've been with him, and he treats me like the queen that I know I am, 'cause I don't want for nothing, thank you very much.

Queenie

If I could sum up the type of work I mean in one word, Queenie, that word would be *communication*. I've learned through my years of dating various men and being in and out of relationships that the main thing is our ability to communicate with our partners. That's the heart and soul of a good relationship. I used to believe that loving someone was enough to justify being in a relationship, but I discovered that love was the icing on the relationship cake. Unless you've got the flour, milk, sugar, and eggs to make the batter and a hot oven to bake it in you don't have a cake to put the icing on, and let's face it, without the cake you've just got a lot of sugar and water—in other words, a sticky sweet mess that tastes good for a while, but if you eat too much of it, like all sweet things, over time you'll get sick of it.

Now the way I see it, in order to make a good relationship cake you have to study the recipes to see what type of cake you're hungry for (meeting people that you're interested in dating); then you have to read the directions to see if you've got all the necessary ingredients (getting to know the person you're interested in, looking at the types of things the two of you might have in common); now after you've assembled everything you need you're ready to make the batter (spend time together getting to know each other); while you're mixing the batter you turn on the oven so it can heat because you want it to be just the right temperature (you may want to test your sexual compatibility at this point); when the batter is just right you pour it in the pan and stick it in the oven to bake (at this point you'll want to see if the relationship can develop into something more). After the cake is done you're ready to decorate it with icing (now we're talking about love).

I know this is a rather long description, but I think it fits because at each step in this process we're dealing with communication. How can I know someone unless I know something about how he may fit into my world or how I fit into his? The only way I'm going to get this information is through communication. I started to bake a lot of cakes in the past, only to discover that I didn't have all the necessary ingredients, or I'd forgotten to turn the oven on, or at the last minute something didn't go right and the cake fell, leaving me with a gooey, half-baked mess on my hands. I'm slowly learning to bake my relationship cakes with respect and trust as the main ingredients and love as the icing. Now I know that a lot of us aren't into baking cakes or anything else for that matter, but I believe the same rules apply. I believe that loving someone and seeing if that person loves you is worth the time and energy.

Personally, sis, I've seen your kitchen and it don't look like you do a whole lot of baking or cooking period, but I like the way you laid out the idea of having to build on a relationship. But it's like I told you, I like variety—I guess you could call me more of a muffin person, little cakes with lots of taste.

Zoey

There's nothing wrong with short-term relationships or even one-night stands, Zoey, but we have to be clear with ourselves and the other person about our agenda. I've noticed that a lot of sisters give lip service to wanting to date but what they want is a committed long-term relationship. It's like they look in the cookbook and decide they're going to make cookies because they want something easy and sweet. But what they really want is a cake and they're disappointed that the cookies don't look or taste like a cake.

I may be wrong here, but it sounds to me like you're saying that the sisters are the ones responsible for making things work out. What I want to know is while we're slaving in the kitchen what are the brothers doing?

Ella

It may sound as if the sisters are doing all the work, Ella, but the brothers have to be willing to throw on an apron and get flour on their hands too. I do think that we as women have to be clear about what we want, because that's the only way we can make choices for ourselves. That's why I said and will continue to say that communication is the key ingredient. Oftentimes sisters allow the brothers to do all the baking—make all of the choices—and then we get upset when they decide to eat their cake too.

Good communication involves talking and listening. I forgot that last part in my first relationship, and I lost six years because I forgot to pay attention to one of the key ingredients. Gracie said that it took her two tries to get the cake that she wanted, and while it doesn't taste exactly like the cake she had before, she enjoys enough of the flavor to continue eating.

Well, I think I'm gonna go for the measured commitment approach. I'm gonna give him measure for measure what he gives me. I get tired of always puttin' myself out only to lose it all in the end.

Ella

You know what they say, Ella, you only get as good as you give. You don't give nothin', chances are you ain't gonna get nothin' either.

Jonie

Yeah, well, all I can say is I'm damn tired of giving all the time. I'll just have to take my chances. I went with this one guy for three months, I mean I really poured my heart and soul into the thing, only to find out the dude was married and just stringing me along. And to top it off, I found out later the fool was using drugs. Even if he wasn't married I wouldn't have put up with that mess. For whatever reason I just keep picking losers. Maybe it's my karma 'cause for whatever reason I just don't seem to be able to get it right.

Ella

Maybe it's like sis said, Ella, you just don't take the time to bake your cake till it's done.

Stella

That's why I say that it's important to get information by way of communication for ourselves when we look at having a relationship. I don't think we purposely go into a relationship knowing that we'll get hurt. Maybe I'm naive but I just don't think hurting is our primary goal. But sometimes I think we get so carried away (Lord knows I've been in that boat) that we forget what's important to us in the long term and we start making the icing before we even decide on what type of cake we want to eat.

Before I got with Willie, and I ain't proud of this, mind you, I was with a married man. Brother man was good to me and Summer, but I knew it wasn't gonna go nowhere 'cause he told me up front that he was married and wasn't plannin' on leavin' his wife and kids. I played the game for a while because I felt like I wanted somebody in my life. But after a while it started feelin' like I was gettin' the scraps from the table of life, so I broke it off. But then I met Willie and we've been eatin' off the same plate so to speak ever since.

Queenie

Personally I think affairs are dangerous, but I also know that for a variety of reasons people get caught up in them from time to time. But again, communication plays a role here too. If we know in the beginning that the guy is married we can adjust our expectations accordingly, but if we don't know he's married we're left with a lot of hurt and pain.

Take my word for it, there's gonna be pain either way, 'cause he can walk away intact anytime he wants, but you've still got to deal with yourself. When I found out my first husband was having an affair, it like to killed me. I knew we were in trouble, but I just didn't figure it would get to that, know what I mean? I was so mad at him till I tracked her down and gave her a piece of my mind. She was young and told me that she didn't know he was married, and I believed her, 'cause knowing him she probably didn't. Then I took him back. He never admitted that he was wrong, in fact he just wanted to forget it, but I couldn't forget it so we ended up parting ways. Yes ma'am, relationships are work, that's for sure, but when you got somebody who's willing to work with you it makes all the difference in the world.

Gracie

What I enjoy most about my relationship with LaShay is the fact that she's real romantic. I used to think that romance was something that people only wrote about in books, but being with that woman has really allowed me to explore and enjoy the softer side of myself. She not only communicates her feelings for me through words; she shows me in little ways that she loves me and values our relationship by what she does, and I'm not just talking about sex either. Although that's pretty damn good too.

Nonie

Gosh! Even Nonie with her li'l pretty young self can get it right. Maybe I'm just on the wrong side of the relationship fence.

Ella

Come on, Ella. You know better than that. Things are good between me and Shay because we work at them. Lesbian couples have some of the same issues and problems that straight couples have when it comes to relationships. Honey, let's face it—being together requires time and energy, I don't care who you are.

Nonie

You're right, girlfriend. I guess I just got a little carried away with feeling sorry for myself.

Ella

That's a good point, Nonie. I also like what you were saying about how our communication doesn't always happen with words. We communicate a great deal in our interactions with our partners. In the beginning of a relationship we depend heavily on our verbal skills to give and get needed information, but as we get to know a person better we start using different forms of communication in order to let our partner know how we feel about certain things.

I know just what you're talking about, but that's how my relationship started with DeWayne. We met at our cousin's barbecue, and DeWayne swears he started talking to me 'cause I gave him "the look." Now we tease each other with "the look." Like he'll come home from work, and if I give him that little sideways glance, he'll know I'm in the mood to mess around. And what really cracks me up is when he's in the mood he'll say something like "Baby, I'm giving you 'the look,' " and he starts winking at me. So it's like we started communicating without words right off the bat.

Jonie

I like that, Jonie, and you're right too. Sometimes our communication can start out nonverbal. But it's still important to get that verbal thing going on too.

Jonie, you got DeWayne givin' you looks and Willie lets me know he wants some by helpin' me with the dishes. I can tell just as good when Willie's in the mood to get some, 'cause he'll hang around the kitchen and start helpin' me to clean up and we have what I call warm chatter. You know, making small talk while I wash the dishes and he dries them and puts them away. I used to fuss with him when he first started doing it, 'cause it seemed like that was the only time he'd help out round the house. But after a while I started likin' it, 'cause I figured out that it was his way of being romantic.

Queenie

Go 'head on, Miss Queenie, with your old self, talkin' about romance. I didn't know you had it in you at your age.

Ella

Girl, you better hush. I may be older but I done forgot more in the department of romance then you'll ever get the chance to learn. We may not do all that fancy stuff but we get it on and age ain't got a thing to do with gittin' some good lovin', take my word for it. There may be snow on the roof, but there's still fire in the furnace and my old man knows just how to stoke it to make it burn.

Queenie

You tell her, Queenie. These young mamas ain't got nothing on us—we invented the rules and they're just learning how to play the game. But I have to agree with sis too, until we start learning how to talk about what we want and need in the kitchen, we ain't never going make it to the bedroom.

Zoey

All I can say to that, Zoey, is amen.

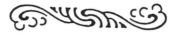

SAAB
(SINGLE, ATTRACTIVE, AVAILABLE & BLACK)

I've been preoccupied for days now with the thought of Dave's leaving. It's not that I'm surprised. At the very beginning of our brief but intense six-month relationship he told me that he had accepted a teaching position in Boston and would be leaving in the fall. I remember thanking the Goddess for allowing me to meet an honest up-front man—someone who revealed his plans in April on our second date, when it became obvious to both of us that we shared a very strong mutual sexual attraction toward each other. This is perfect, I thought; I don't have the time or energy in my life for a drawn-out romantic relationship. In fact, I had become so accustomed to my single status in the past three and half years that I even bought a Saab (which I proudly told everyone stood for Single, Attractive, Available & Black) to symbolize acceptance of my relationship status.

I met Dave at a friend's dinner party, and while it was clear at the time that we shared a love of the theater, books, a dry sense of humor, travel, and mutual friends, we didn't get together right away because he was going off to Europe for three months and I was headed out on a lengthy book tour. We exchanged phone numbers and agreed to keep in touch. In all honesty I didn't really expect to hear from him again—after all, three months is a long time—and at this stage in my life I was used to meeting guys, exchanging pleasantries and phone numbers, and never hearing from them again. So needless to say I was fairly surprised and somewhat intrigued when I picked up my phone messages four months later to get a message from him, inviting me to dinner and a movie. We never made it to the movie; we spent our first date getting to know each other, talking and laughing over a leisurely dinner in a cozy Seattle café. I found myself comfortably gazing into his warm brown eyes as he shared with me his dream of someday becoming the dean of a small college. I listened halfheartedly as he told me of his experiences living and teaching in different parts of the world, while letting my mind wonder what it would be like to have him kiss me. I wanted him sexually, and a kiss from him would tell me if he wanted me too.

I love kissing; it's fun. In fact, next to whooping and hollering with my friends when we're watching basketball, kissing is my favorite participatory sport. Through a lot of trial and error over the years I've discovered the best way to assess a person's sexual personality is by his manner of kissing. A deep, probing kiss is a signal of someone who wants to know you inside and out; little bites on the lips between kisses are a signal of sexual hunger, and you get to be the main course; little pecks on the lips accompanied by warm close hugs are a signal that closeness is more important than sex; and a quick kiss on a closed mouth means forget it, sex isn't even an option.

I found myself hoping that Dave was deep and hungry enough to leave me weak and starved. I wasn't disappointed. Dave walked me to my car after our two-hour dinner, and as I fished in my purse for my keys, I felt his arms slip around my waist and, looking up, I encountered his lips zeroing in on mine; the sweet, passionate hunger in his kiss was so deep that I felt like butter, creamy, smooth, and ready to spread. Dave's kiss definitely told me what I wanted to know, that he was as hungry as I was, and if this kiss was the appetizer it wouldn't be long before I got to sample the full meal deal.

Driving home from that first date I had the impression that we would be good together sexually. So on our second date, when Dave told me about his plans to move to Boston in the fall, I mentally relaxed my usual rule of having six dates before sex. And on our fourth date I discovered that my initial impression of sex with Dave was right on. After all, I reasoned to myself, I'm only interested in cookies (an easy, brief encounter), and this man was perfect: handsome, fun, was attracted to me, had a life, and most important, he would be leaving—there's no chance to get attached. After all, I had plans of my own—work, writing, travel—and I didn't need or want attachments at this point in my life, or so I thought. In the beginning of our relationship, the thought that he would be leav-

ing stayed in the front of my mind, as a steady reminder not to get too close emotionally.

But I hadn't counted on this man to physically and
emotionally pull out all the stops. He cooked sexually
like a pro, and after spending three and a half years
on a sexual starvation diet I ate with gusto. Lying in
bed, caressing his chest, running my fingers down his
well-muscled stomach and enjoying the fine essence
of his maleness, I forgot that I was only interested in
cookies, and my mind played the unforgivable game
of baking a tempting marble cake (long-term relationship), icing and all. He was so easy to be with, we
laughed and played well together . . . what if . . . I
found myself wondering as we lay side by side cud-
dling. But there had been steady reminders all along
the way that Dave would be leaving: trips to the East
Coast to look for housing, telephone conferences with
school officials, selling off different household items
because it wouldn't make sense to haul them across
country, and the excitement in his voice whenever he
talked about his new position.

Zoey had tried to warn me early on when I first told
her of my plans for a brief encounter with Dave. "You
know, sis, some of us are born to be attached, and
some of us can do with or without it. Just remember,
sex is like food: some folks just want an appetizer,
other folks need a full meal in order to be satisfied,
and then some can make do with dessert. Now I been
knowing you for a long time and you say that you
want dessert, but watch out 'cause personally I think
you're more of a full-meal person, if you take my
meaning."

Of course I assured Zoey that I knew just what I wanted, and Dave fit the bill perfectly. But slowly, without fully recognizing it, my agenda started to change, and maybe that change had to do with the time we spent together. Because of our busy schedules, we burned up the phone lines with our nightly calls and generally saved our weekends to be together. But the time we did spend with each other—attending concerts on the Seattle Pier, going to author readings at the Elliott Bay Bookstore, watching foreign films at the Harvard Exit Theater, enjoying cozy dinners at the Coastal Kitchen Cafe, and taking long, leisurely, hand-in-hand strolls on Broadway, peeking in shop windows playing "If I had a million dollars"—had something to do with the change I was experiencing. I do know that the primary factor in moving me to change my taste from dessert to the full meal happened in the bedroom, because no matter how our evening started it ended with passionate sex. Dave was full of surprises in as well as out of the bedroom. He would tease my erotic senses with soft sensuous wordplay as a sweet interlude, while massaging me with his masterful strategic touch. Then without a hint of warning he would move from a gentle, sensitive, intuitive lover to being passionately forceful, his predatory male strength bending my mind and body to his will. I loved it all. Dave openly invited my sexual fantasies while tenderly soothing my fears through words of acceptance and sensitive touch. More than any other man I've ever been with, Dave welcomed and encouraged my desire to be playful as well as romantic with sex.

"We have great sex together," I commented one afternoon as we lay cuddled together after a particularly enjoyable time. "No, baby," he replied, in a voice filled with contentment, "what we make is love. We make great love together." My ears and mind must be playing tricks on me, I thought as I drifted in and out of a dream state, curled up close, my head on his chest, lulled to sleep by the rhythm of his strong, steady heartbeat.

Later that evening, at home in my bed, I allowed myself to retrieve the memory of our afternoon together, and with the memory came the statement "We make great love together"; could it be that Dave's thoughts about our togetherness had changed? Maybe he was baking a cake too. I smiled to myself at the thought. After all, he must have realized how emotionally loaded the *L* word can be in any situation, and to use it at the beginning, middle, or end of sex was truly significant in my book. I had chosen to be carefully guarded in my language with him, purposely not using emotionally loaded words in order to keep my perspective clear. But here he was using the *L* word, without fear or trepidation. I gave a little thought to the fact that my ears might have deceived me—after all I had been meaning to have them checked for some time—but I was ninety-nine percent sure that Dave had said the word *love*. I had been sleepy, not deaf. Because I wanted to believe in my growing fantasy of our lasting long-term togetherness based on the use of one word, the *L* word, by him, I immersed myself in a secure cocoon of firm denial. He wouldn't have said it if he didn't mean it, I told myself over and over, trying to squelch what I perceived to be my unfounded fears that maybe I was mistaken in what I had heard Dave say. Fate was fate, as far as I was concerned, and who was I to argue with the love gods? This man was in love with me, I just knew it.

There was a movie not too long ago entitled *Reality Bites*—well, I'm here to testify that reality not only bites; it will sink its sharp, ugly teeth into your flesh and chew with the vigor of a rabid dog. I felt the ravished bite of reality on our next weekend together when Dave announced that he was going to be spending the following week in a hotel because the movers would be coming on Thursday in order to move his stuff. Wait just a damn minute! my mind screamed as I lay quietly next to him in bed. He's playing some kind of sadistic trick on me trying to get a reaction. Hmm, that's totally out of character for him, I reasoned as I waited patiently for him to yell "Gotcha!" But the gotcha never came. "I've been thinking," Dave said, crawling over me, stopping long enough to plant a quick kiss on my numb lips on his way to the bathroom to shower. "Since you like San Francisco so much, why don't we spend our last weekend together there? Honey, are you coming? The water's just the way you like it." I mumbled something about being sleepy, and rolled over to muffle my sobs of disappointment in the pillow.

It's Monday, Dave leaves on Thursday, and I can't seem to think about anything else. As a matter of survival I've started creating lists again. I declined the trip to San Francisco in favor of spending the last few days together at a nice downtown hotel. I have this little game I play whenever I feel confused about a situation in my life, when I don't know what to think: I just stop thinking and revert to automatic pilot. So on our last weekend together I spent the entire time re-creating the emotional boundaries that I had abandoned much too quickly. Dave attributed my lack of playful enthusiasm to my sadness over his leaving, and because he was partially right I didn't bother to correct his assumption.

Leaking tears in the office bathroom, losing sleep, ignoring chocolate—I thought I had given up these signs of misery for Lent. I needed comfort, a release from the feelings and thoughts that threatened to overwhelm me, and I needed that comfort now.

"Hello, Zoey, it's me."

"What's the matter, baby? What time is it? Who's in jail?"

"It's me, Zoey, sis; it's twelve a.m. and nobody's in jail. I'm hurting and I need to talk."

"Okay, baby, okay, just give me a minute to collect myself. This damn head rag slipped down over my eyes, and I can't see a blessed thing. My head's gonna look a mess in the mornin', and I just got it done today. . . . What's goin' on, sweetcakes? Are you sick? Do you need to go to the ER? Where in the hell did I leave my keys?"

"I'm okay physically, but Dave's leaving for Boston in two days, and I'm having a tough time handling it. You were right—I tried to make a full meal out of cookies, and now my emotional stomach is upset. How could I have been so dumb?"

"Now hold on just a minute there, sweetcakes. Don't

go being so hard on yourself. You're a lot of things—mainly hardheaded—but you're not dumb. Now settle down and tell me what's goin' on."

I heard Zoey exhale the smoke from her cigarette and mentally pictured her sitting on the side of the bed cradling the phone with her shoulder as she stared straight ahead listening intently to my tale of woe. I knew that she would listen for as long as I needed to talk.

". . . So when he said we made great love together, I just automatically jumped to the conclusion that he somehow meant for us to be together long-term. You would think that I'd know better—after all, I'm a therapist, I have training in communication—but I clearly missed the boat on this one. I feel so foolish. . . . Zoey! Zoey, are you there?"

"I'm here, baby. I'm just listening is all. I was thinking, a kiss together with some good sex can be a dangerous combination when you're hungry. And you were starved, so it makes good sense that you would want to eat. You got a little carried away, but that doesn't mean you did anything wrong."

"I should have known better."

"You did know better, but that's not the issue. The issue is a matter of the heart. Dave touched your heart, and I'm willing to bet that you started baking that cake you always talk about long before he said the *L* word. You're used to being in love, that's what you know, so that's what you do, and last time I checked being in love ain't no sin."

"How do you do it, Zoey? You have little affairs all

the time, and you never seem to get caught up in the love thing."

"It's not that I don't love them, baby, 'cause I do, in my own way. I may not fall in love with a capital *L*, because loving with the small *l* suits my needs better. I love the time I spend with the person I'm with, but I know that it's me doing the loving and since it's mine to give, I can give it at will. But just like I give it I can take it with me when I go. My mama taught me how to leave a long time ago, when she took me and walked out on my sorry-ass abusive father. Sometimes I think I learned that lesson a little too well, 'cause now I leave whenever a situation looks like it might be painful, and that includes emotional pain. I ain't saying what I do is right or wrong but that's what I know and that's what I do. Sometimes I even wish I could stick it out, but I ain't never been one to gain through pain, even my own. I don't have to guard or protect my feelings when it comes to love, sex, or anything else when I'm with somebody because I know how to walk. But just because that works for me it don't mean it'll work for you or anybody else."

"Zoey."

"Yeah, sweetcakes."

"Thanks."

"You're welcome, baby. You know I'm always goin' to be here for you. Now let's get some sleep, 'cause I'm definitely gonna have to wrestle with this head in the mornin'. And, sis."

"Yeah, Zoey?"

"I love you."

"I love you too, Zoey. Good night."

Outside of my parents, nobody could call me baby and mean it the way Zoey does. And because I know she does love me, I could take her words of wisdom to heart—she never steers me wrong. I lay in bed and thought about our conversation; even though I didn't want to admit it, Zoey was right, bless her tough old hide, about my knowing how to fall in love, because that's what I knew how to do. I wanted to believe that I was grown enough to love 'em and leave 'em, as they say, without the emotional baggage that comes with attachments, but my feelings of sadness, hurt, and loss told me different. Emotionally, I was carrying around a whole set of Louis Vuitton luggage and all Dave had was a knapsack. Having watched my parents love and tough it out with each other for forty-plus years of their fifty-three year marriage taught me how to embrace the fire of love even during the stormy times. I knew from my divorce that some storms were strong enough to blow out the flame, leaving a feeling of cold hardness to fill the void. In my case the divorce blew out the flame but the embers were still warm and ready to flicker at the first sign of a breeze. Being unaware of my nature at the start of our relationship, I could now better understand how having Dave speak the *L* word was the breeze I needed to ignite my passionately warm embers. Understanding all of this didn't make Dave's leaving any easier for me, but it did make me aware of the fact that all relationships, sexual or otherwise, are in fact based on a degree of negotiation with your partner as well as with yourself. In the beginning I was clear that I was only interested in a sexual relationship, and that's the contract that I emotionally communicated. However, when I discovered that sex wasn't going to be enough, I changed the contract but neglected to share that piece of information.

I don't care what anybody says, I was taught that sex outside of marriage is wrong, and what you've just said kind of proves that point. If you had gone into that relationship with the understanding that it would end somewhere positive you wouldn't have gotten hurt.

Roxy

You can't be serious, Roxy—people have sex all the time with or without marriage. And besides, being married doesn't guarantee you anything these days, all you have to do is look around at all the people, men and women, involved in extramarital affairs.

Jonie

Actually the only thing that I can see that sis didn't pay attention to here is her feelings. Like she said, she moved from a spoken contract to an unspoken contract without letting her friend in on it.

Zoey

You're right, Zoey. When I changed directions I forgot that I wasn't the only person on the train. Marriage was never my intent—I wanted a sexual partner. And as good as the sex was, marriage wouldn't have entered the picture because I'm just not ready to take that step.

You know, I wonder how men do it—they don't seem to have the same hang-ups that women have about sex without marriage. They can move from one person to another without giving it a second thought.

Ella

I think that men do have some of the same thoughts that we have about sex, but the difference is they get more societal permission to enjoy their sexual activities without guilt. Actually there are some women who can allow themselves to enjoy sex without the benefit of having a relationship, but I discovered that I'm not one of them. I tried it and discovered that I've still got a lot to learn about myself and brief sexual encounters.

Well, I'll be your teacher, because I've been in so many dysfunctional relationships until I don't even have a clue as to what a normal healthy relationship looks like anymore. I know what's supposed to happen but it never does and I'm sick of trying to be honest. So the only relationships I'm interested in anymore are those of a sexual nature. All I want these days is good, clean, safe, unencumbered sex.

Ella

Ella, you're just too choosy is all, and you got a chip on your shoulder. How you expect to even find somebody if all you want them for is sex?

Queenie

That may be true, but at least I'm not walking around crying the blues 'cause things didn't work out.

Ella

You better watch yourself, girlfriend, 'cause just when you say that up jumps the devil. You know it don't pay to play with Mother Nature, 'cause she'll grab you every time. Look what happened to sis.

Cyree

You know, Ella, I'm a lot like you when it comes to brief encounters, but I think my situation has more to do with fear of being hurt then anything else. I was in a long-term relationship at one point—the guy loved me and I knew I loved him too—but I didn't know it till it was too late to do anything about it. He was a good man, somebody I could trust and care about, but I was so used to being hurt emotionally by guys till it never dawned on me that he wouldn't try to hurt me. I kept waitin' for him to mess up somehow, and when he didn't mess up, I started distrusting myself and became afraid of hurting him. Pretty soon he got tired of waiting and ended up marrying somebody else.

Zoey

Gosh, Zoey, I never knew that. I just thought that you were a player. You know, like a lot of the guys, who just don't take love seriously.

Ella

Well, you never knew it, because I don't talk about it. Yeah, I play around a lot, because like you said, I was one of those that cried the blues, and discovered that I didn't like it. So it's not that I don't trust guys as much as I don't trust myself not to get hurt. Like I told sis, I learned to walk away from pain a long time ago, and I ain't gonna lie, sometimes walkin' away has saved me from a lot of grief, but that one time, hangin' in there might've served me better. I guess sometimes we just have to be willing to take a chance, and trust them as well as trusting ourselves.

Zoey

My problem is how do you know? How do you know when to trust and when to let go? I've gotten stung so many times believing the hype that men lay on you till it's just easier not to believe. I'm so used to them sayin' what they want you to hear until I just quit listenin'. I've been in sis's situation, and gettin' left at the altar was the final straw for me. After that I just said to myself, Girlfriend, you're never gonna go through this again.

Ella

Ella, I didn't know you were left at the altar. When did that happen?

Stella

It happened a few years back. I don't know if you all remember LaMar—he was in the service. Well, I was head over heels in love with that man. I mean, he promised me the sun, moon, and stars plus a few things in between. He kept telling me that he loved me and he wanted to settle down and get married and he wanted me to have his babies. I bought the hype lock, stock, and barrel. We even picked out rings and talked about where we'd live. Then he got stationed in Texas and I got phone calls and letters for a while, but I noticed that the calls and letters never mentioned anything about setting a date. I had even planned to move down there so I could be close by him 'cause he said he was going to be in Texas a couple of years. But then when I told him that he started actin' funny, saying things like "Baby, I really want you here but you wouldn't like it," and stuff like that. After that the calls and letters really slowed down. The last time I talked to him he said that he wasn't really ready for the marriage thing, that his life was too unsettled right now. Well, honey, that was the last call I made and the last time I talked to him. And like I said, after that experience I told myself no more for me. Here I was all ready to stick with this man till death do us part—I'm just glad I found out about him before it got that far.

Ella

You know, Ella, I do remember you talkin' about LaMar, but then you stopped talkin' about him and I just thought that maybe you had kicked him to the curb, 'cause I'm so used to you goin' from one guy to the next without a vacation in between till I just chalked him up to another one of your tribe.

Jonie

Yeah, well, he's a long-gone memory now.

Ella

You're awful quiet over there, sis. Still thinkin' about Dave?

Zoey

Yeah, Zoey, I was thinking about him, but I was also thinking about this conversation we're having. I think you and Ella have raised some pretty interesting points. I mean, how do we know when to trust our instincts about love? When is it okay to believe and not believe what we're hearing from someone we're involved with at the moment? You wanted to trust but you didn't and Ella wanted to trust and she did, and I wanted to believe in a miracle, and we all got hurt, so what's the answer?

Well, I don't know about you two, but from here on in I'm doing it my way. I'm just gonna trust myself not to believe the hype. If I don't get too close in the beginning I can't get distracted by the BS. I may lose out once in a while but at least I'll be the one in control.

Ella

I don't know, Ella, that was my agenda too, remember, and I still got caught up in the emotional stuff. I wanted to keep my distance but it just didn't work out. I think it comes down to what Zoey told me before: relationships and sex are like food; some of us can make do with appetizers, some of us need the full-meal deal, and some of us only want dessert. But the real challenge comes in knowing just how hungry we are at the time.

Well, as for myself, I was pretty sure about my appetite, but I didn't know about his. He wanted the full meal and I didn't think I was hungry enough, mainly because my plate was already full with my own stuff, leftovers from my family background and past relationships. By the time that I discovered that I was hungry for more, boyfriend was gone. I knew my agenda, as you would say, sis, but I didn't want to take the time to know his agenda.

Zoey

You know I think it's more a matter of steppin' out on faith. I guess I just got lucky with Phil. It took me a while to know and trust loving him because of my first two marriages. But I noticed right away that he was different. For one thing he wasn't as exciting to me as my first two husbands—of course I don't even count my first husband because we were both so young; I was nineteen and he was twenty-one and I just wanted to be married 'cause all of my friends were doing it. But Carl, he was this big hotshot accountant, working for this firm, climbing the corporate ladder, you know—all the perks, as they say. But he was so wrapped up in his own game until he just didn't have room for me or anybody else. I was just another trophy, as a sign of his success. But Phil has always been real. Because we taught at the same school I really had a chance to observe him on a day-to-day basis, and I liked what I saw, the way he interacted with other people, the way he was with the kids at school, firm but gentle. I just got a real good chance to see and know his nature, and from watching him in those situations it gave me a good idea of what he'd be like with me.

Gracie

Maybe that's a strong key to this whole puzzle, Gracie. Taking the time to really get to know the person we want to be involved with on a day-to-day basis. I spent time with Dave, but it wasn't extended periods of time, I liked the picture I created of us, but that picture wasn't fully developed. I wanted him to see and want the picture I had created without thinking about the fact that he had created his own picture of us.

You know, sis, that sounds all well and good, but I don't really think there is one answer. I just think we all get caught up emotionally from time to time. The only key I have is me—I know what I'm about and I've come to accept it. Like I said before, what I do and how I do it ain't everybody's cup of tea and it ain't right or wrong, it's just me. I may change somewhere down the road but for right now, I just have to do what fits.

Zoey

Well, a man is really gonna have to show me some-thing before I put my heart out on a limb again. It's a shame to say it, but the next guy is gonna have to wipe out all the doubts that those before him put in my mind.

                                    Ella

I guess it just boils down to being willing to take a chance. But I think we stand a better chance if we do a couple of things first. Like Zoey says, we've got to know ourselves well enough to know what we want in a relationship, and like Gracie said, we have to be willing to investigate the person we're interested in being involved with long-term.

What about your approach of believing in miracles, sis?

                                    Jonie

Well, I guess you're right, Jonie. We could believe in miracles too. But sometimes miracles need a little help.

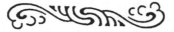

EMBRACING THE FIRE

I recently attended a friend's wedding. It was a beautiful affair in the park, with flowers in bloom, trees towering overhead, bright radiant sun beaming down from a clear cornflower blue sky. It was the kind of day that seduces me into staying in Seattle despite the overabundance of gray sunless days that seem to fill most of the calendar year. LaSharon was beautiful, in her cream-colored beaded afternoon wedding dress and garden hat, standing next to Lionel in his black tux. Theirs was the first wedding I had attended in years—as a matter of fact, this was the first wedding I had attended since my own fifteen years ago. Knowing my aversion to this type of ceremony, LaSharon had asked me to come as my gift to her: "I need you there, girlfriend. You've always been there for me during the rough times, and now I want you there to help me celebrate my good times. Your being at my wedding would mean the world to me. Consider it your gift to me and Lionel, okay? Do this one thing for me."

I promised to think about it, but deep down inside I knew I wouldn't let LaSharon down. I had watched her grow from an awkward, tough-talking adolescent woman-child to a mature woman in her own right. We had met at the start of my career, when I was called in to do some work with LaSharon, who was involved in a severely dysfunctional lifestyle. LaSharon's mother had died from a drug overdose, and at age fourteen LaSharon, the youngest of five, was being raised by her grandmother, a sweet, kindhearted woman who shared with her granddaughter a love of alcohol and didn't have the energy or good health to keep up with a budding teenager who had witnessed more in her fourteen years than most of us see in a lifetime. While in her mother's care LaSharon had been introduced to drugs and alcohol at age twelve, and she had run away from home and lived on the streets for a couple of years before coming to the attention of authorities. I met LaSharon after her first go-round in a recovery program, and throughout our years together I would become her anchor as she struggled through several more recovery programs, dropped out of school, had two children removed from her custody, and was involved in countless abusive relationships. At age eighteen LaSharon disappeared from sight, and I moved on, changing jobs and directions in my life, and thinking about her often.

One day about two years ago I received a phone call at my office—it was LaSharon. She had tracked me down at my place of employment and wanted to have lunch and bring me up-to-date, as she put it, on what was happening in her life. I invited her to my office,

but she declined, stating that this wasn't about ther-
apy, it was about friendship, and she had something
to tell me. I agreed, and we met at a local deli a week
later. I didn't recognize her at first. She was dressed in
a lovely spring dress, with her hair cut short and fram-
ing her expertly made-up face; she hardly resembled
the sagging-blue-jeaned, Nike-and-backward-base-
ball-cap-wearing teenager I had known for so many
years. Over salads and iced tea LaSharon updated me
on her life. Her grandmother had died from a stroke,
which had thrown LaSharon into a downward spiral
back to drugs and alcohol. She had tried to live with
an older sister, but there was too much conflict, so she
went back to living on the streets. After nearly dying
from an overdose, LaSharon went back into recovery
at a two-year facility, where she met Lionel, who, as
she described him, was determined to get his life together. LaSharon said that counseling, attending NA
(Narcotics Anonymous) and AA (Alcoholics Anonymous), and meeting Lionel saved her life. She com-
pleted her high school courses and started taking
classes at the local community college. At the time of
our meeting she had been clean and sober for two
years and had been working as a receptionist at the
telephone company for nine months. She and Lionel
were living together and he too was still clean, attending school, and working for a local construction firm.
LaSharon told me how much she loved Lionel and
how his love of her had kept her strong, and like him,
she was determined to get her life together.

Then she told me her big news, that she and Lionel
were getting married and she wanted to invite me to

their wedding. "You know, girlfriend, you told me something a long time ago that's stuck with me. You said that while I might be my mother's daughter, I didn't have to live my mother's life. I guess it took a while for the message to sink in, but I'm glad it finally did." That's when she invited me to her wedding. After congratulating her on her many successes, I added quickly, "I don't know, LaSharon. I haven't attended a wedding in years, but I want to give you and Lionel a really special gift. What would you like?"

"I've told Lionel all about you, and we both agree that the only gift we want from you is for you to come to our wedding," she stated firmly as she kissed me on the cheek and gathered her things, preparing to walk back to her downtown office.

As I walked back uptown to my own office I thought about LaSharon with just a tinge of pride, and I must admit a bit of worry. My pride was in how much work she had put into turning her life around. I had watched LaSharon go through recovery a number of times only to crumble whenever life became too stressful. I was proud of her for setting her sights on a goal and working toward it with firm determination. I worried because LaSharon was still her mother's daughter, and while she'd had numerous experiences with abusive relationships, she didn't have a model that I knew about for a healthy relationship. I believed her when she said that she was going to turn her life around, but I worried because her goal was love, and I knew that love could be stressful.

I remember, as though it was yesterday, being called to the second recovery center that LaSharon had been placed in, because she was in danger of being dismissed for breaking the rule of sneaking out after curfew and being caught downtown with a group of her old friends. LaSharon was brought back to the center by the police, who in trying to be helpful told her that she really needed to shape up, that she'd never grow up to find love and happiness if she kept hanging out on street corners doing drugs. Being in one of her angry self-destructive modes, she told me that she didn't believe in love, it was all Hollywood hype that got put in TV movies. She said her mother had told her that she herself didn't believe in love, 'cause it didn't pay enough, and that if anybody told LaSharon that they loved her it was a lie. I told La-Sharon that her mother was mistaken about love and she didn't have to live her mother's life, that she could in fact write her own script for her life. Sitting on the side of LaSharon's bed in the small room where she had been confined, I stroked her head in my lap as she sobbed tears of anger and hurt. Trying to ease her pain, I gently explained that sometimes our mothers pack our emotional suitcases in a fit of reckless desperation with hand-me-downs from their own life experiences, in the hope that we'll grow into and get some use out of them. Often our mothers forget that we need room in that suitcase to pack our own stuff and a few new things (our experiences) that we might collect along the way. Not feeling really sure that LaSharon was listening at the time, but wanting to soothe some of her fears, I encouraged her to remember that she wasn't her mother and she was old enough now to pack her own emotional suitcases, because this was her life.

As I watched LaSharon and Lionel exchange their personal vows of love and commitment, my thoughts turned to my own emotional baggage about these issues. I had definitely done some rearranging and repacking over the years. Momi had packed everything—love, trust, commitment, loyalty, and sex—in neat tidy piles, coordinating, and folding each item just so, making sure that each piece had a place in my life, leaving just enough room to avoid unwanted creases and wrinkles. And while my bags looked well kept and neat throughout my adolescence, I discovered as a woman that Momi had forgotten to leave room for my life experiences. I had tried on many of the things that Momi had packed for me only to find that I had outgrown them (my marriage) or the color wasn't right (trust). And some things I found that I liked, but I got tired of the wrinkles and creases that forever needed pressing (love). I also added items to my suitcase that I knew Momi wouldn't approve of because they would take up space without adding value—like divorce, casual sexual relationships, affairs of the heart, and long-term relationships that wouldn't end in marriage—experiences that I had in my life that weren't planned, but I needed to make room to carry them too. Where Momi packed with neat precision, choosing each item with care, I took a more casual, haphazard approach and reverted back to her methods only in times of emotional confusion.

I had steered clear of attending weddings because

they evoked memories of how much I missed loving and being loved by someone special. While I could manage outwardly on a day-to-day basis to convince myself that my mother's emotional luggage for a relationship was much too heavy to carry, I inwardly felt a twinge of panic thinking about my own method of packing as I watched this couple unite in marriage, declaring their love and affection for each other. After all, I was my mother's daughter, and as much as I tried to hide it, I could feel the words that they spoke start to peel away that fragile layer of haphazard comfort I had worked so hard to put in place. I recognized that I was indeed my mother's daughter, a strong believer in long-term love, or as Zoey so tactfully put it, I needed the full-meal deal in order to feel fulfilled. I could make do with the cookies of short-term affairs, and I was even learning the ropes of having safe casual sex. I got the hang of setting firm emotional boundaries after my relationship with Dave, by following Ella's practice of hearing but not listening to the hype and by choosing men who always had one foot out the door. But even with all the practice in the world, I was still my mother's daughter, and I would have to come to terms with my need to love and be loved. I had rewritten my life script, just as I had encouraged LaSharon to rewrite hers, and I would no doubt rewrite it again many times. But unlike LaSharon, I had found some useful items in the suitcase that Momi had packed for me, and believing in love, even if I decided to wear it differently, was one of the items that I chose to keep forever and ever.

As I passed through Lionel and LaSharon's receiving line, LaSharon hugged me, planted a sweet kiss on my cheek, and whispered, "Don't forget to invite me to your wedding." I whispered back, "It's a promise."

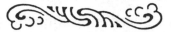

EPILOGUE

"Hi, hon. I know it's been a while since you've heard from me. But I've finally gotten settled in. Between figuring out class assignments, meeting faculty members, getting to know my students, and making my apartment livable I've been up to my eyebrows in work. From what I've seen so far, Boston is a pretty nice place. I was wondering how you'd feel about flying out for the holiday weekend. I miss you, babe. Give me a call and let's talk. My number is . . ."

I replayed the phone message three times and each playing evoked different feelings: surprise ("Oh my God, I don't believe it!"); anger ("How dare he, if he thinks I've been just sitting around waiting"); and longing ("I miss you too, babe"). It had been six months since Dave had left, and hearing his voice on my answering machine unleashed all of the thoughts and feeling I had so carefully packed away after his leaving. I poured myself a glass of iced tea, kicked off my shoes, and curled up in my favorite overstuffed chair by the window, all the while debating the pros and cons of returning Dave's call.

I thought of all the disappointment, hurt, and pain I had waded through at the time of his leaving. My entire relationship with Dave had been based on assumptions. I had assumed that we would have a short-term affair and nothing more; then my feelings changed and one word from him ("love") led me to assume his feelings had changed too, and he wouldn't leave. But he left, leaving me to assume that I would never hear from him again. I recognized that in hearing his voice again—telling me about the new situation and telling me he missed me—I was ready to start making a whole new set of assumptions.

As much as I wanted to be with Dave, looking at my old pattern of working from assumptions frightened me into believing I would be hurt again. When I looked at the pro side of our time together, I felt comfortable and at ease. I didn't experience the tension and pressure of trying to be perfect, or strong. I enjoyed laughing, and we laughed a lot together. I appreciated his honesty and candor—we shared spirited conversations that didn't end in arguments. Dave wasn't perfect, but then he never professed to be. I loved being sexual with him, and his attentions to my needs in that area. I could be playful and flirtatious without feeling silly, and most importantly, we shared the same types of humanistic values.

The pros of my internal debate clearly outweighed the cons, and I could almost hear Zoey saying, "So what's the problem, sweetcakes?" The problem for me was that I would have to be willing to give up making assumptions, and trust myself to be openly honest about what I wanted. At this point in my life I knew what I wanted—a loving sexual relationship; after all, I was my mother's daughter, and I was more—I was my own woman as well.

"Hello, Dave . . ."